Reviews for *The GL Diet*, by the same authors:

'Choice is back on the menu'
***The Times*, 14 May 2005**

'At last a book that takes low glycaemic eating to the next level.
Its beauty is in the simplicity and logic of its ideas. I will be
recommending this to all my patients'
Dr Andrew J. Wright, MBChB DRCOG MRCGP DIHom
of The Complete Fatigue Clinic, Bolton, UK

'An easy weight loss plan for life … simpler than
GI and makes better sense …'
***Evening Standard*, 4 January 2005**

'… the GI diet has been superseded by a more
sophisticated version: the glycaemic load (GL) …'
***The Times*, 14 May 2005**

'The GI diet is so last year. Take slimming one stage further with GL,
a more sophisticated way of measuring the impact of food on your
body's energy levels. Now you can love your lunch but still
lose those love handles'
***The Times*, 7 May 2005**

'Try the easy new GL Diet – everyone's talking about it'
***Essentials* (UK), June 2005**

'The Glycaemic Load (GL) is the final part of the jigsaw. Testing for the GI (glycaemic index) of foods is a fantastic breakthrough, but it only gives half the true picture'
Essentials **(South Africa), September 2005**

'A good guide is Nigel Denby's *The GL Diet* ... more useful ... more of a way of eating than a diet book'
***handbag.com*, April 2005**

'Denby's writing is refreshingly clear and easy to understand; there's no high-tech scientific waffle ... it's a simple programme that uses a food selection system based on science, on fact not fad, but most importantly it's been designed to be practical and easy to follow'
***Seven Magazine*, *Sunday Mail* (Cyprus), 3 April 2005**

'The GL diet has been instrumental in helping me get back to my pre-pregnancy weight. It's more than a diet though and has just become a way of life. I've got so much energy and don't have any of those food cravings I'd always associated with diets and healthy eating – I love it!'
Mishal Husain, news anchor,
BBC World News* and *BBC News 24

THE 7-DAY GL DIET

Glycaemic Loading for Easy Weight Loss

Nigel Denby
with Tina Michelucci & Deborah Pyner

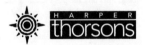

HarperThorsons
An Imprint of HarperCollins*Publishers*
77–85 Fulham Palace Road,
Hammersmith, London W6 8JB

The website address is: www.thorsonselement.com

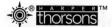

and *HarperThorsons* are trademarks of
HarperCollins*Publishers* Ltd

First published by HarperThorsons 2005

1 3 5 7 9 10 8 6 4 2

© Nigel Denby, Tina Michelucci and Deborah Pyner 2005

Nigel Denby, Tina Michelucci and Deborah Pyner assert the
moral right to be identified as the authors of this work

A catalogue record of this book is
available from the British Library

ISBN-13 978-0-00-722215-5
ISBN-10 0-00-722215-7

Printed and bound in Great Britain by
Clays Ltd, St Ives plc

This publication is meant to be used as a general reference and recipe book to aid weight
loss. As with any weight-loss plan, before commencing we would strongly recommend
that you consult your doctor to see whether it is suitable for you.

While all reasonable care has been taken during the preparation of this book, the
publishers, editors and authors cannot accept responsibility for any
consequences arising from the use of this information.

This book includes reference to nuts and recipes including nuts, nut derivatives and nut
oils. Avoid if you have a known allergic reaction. Pregnant and nursing mothers,
invalids, the elderly, children and babies may be potentially vulnerable to nut
allergies and should therefore avoid nuts, nut derivatives and nut oils.

Contents

Acknowledgements   vii

About the Author   ix

Introduction: The Ultimate Diet   xi

Part I – What is GL?

1   GI and GL Made Simple   3

2   How to Follow the 7-Day GL Diet   12

Part II – Whose Side are You on?

3   It's All in the Mind   27

4   KOKO – Keep on Keeping on   41

5   Every Second Counts   54

Part III – Your 7-Day GL Guides

6   The 7-day Fast and Friendly Plan   61

7   The 7-day Veggie Friendly Plan   76

8   The 7-day Foodie Friendly Plan   107

9   Variety is the Spice of Life   145

Part IV – Living a Low-GL Lifestyle

10 Low-GL Food Lists with Portion Guide   191
11 A Guide to Low-GL Shopping and Eating Out   217
12 Love Your Food *and* Your Body   243

Part V – Further Information

13 The Evidence – Research that Shows   275
    Low-glycaemic Diets Work
14 Your Questions Answered   289

Appendix 1 – A–Z of Low-GL Foods   297
Appendix 2 – Recommended Reading   309

Index   311
Index of Recipes   318

Acknowledgements

Thanks to HarperThorsons and Susanna in particular for her kindness and infectious enthusiasm for the project and for supporting our convictions.

Thanks to our growing band of Diet Freedom Fighters we have gathered from our first book, *The GL Diet*, our website and by word of mouth. We truly hope we have helped you in a small way – it's what motivates us and keeps us going in the wee small hours! Thank you again for your support, kind words, inspiration and honest, constructive feedback, which is invaluable.

And, of course, thanks to our long-suffering partners, families and friends who have been unwavering in their support of our mad working hours, despite our moods and sometimes irrational behaviour. You deserve medals!

Thank you all so very much.

Tina, Deborah and Nigel
xxx

About the Author

Nigel Denby RD BSc Hons trained as a dietician at Glasgow Caledonian University, following an established career in the catering industry. He is a qualified chef and previously owned his own restaurant.

His dietetic career began as a research dietician at the Human Nutrition Research Centre in Newcastle. After a period working as a community dietician, Nigel left the NHS to join Boots Health and Beauty Experience where he led the delivery and training of Boots Nutrition and Weight Management services.

In 2003 Nigel set up his own nutrition consultancy, delivering a clinical service to Hammersmith and Queen Charlotte's Hospital Women's Health Clinic and the International Eating Disorders Centre in Buckinghamshire as well as acting as nutrition consultant for the Childbase Children's Nursery Group.

Nigel also runs his own private practice in Harley Street specializing in weight management, PMS/menopause, irritable bowel syndrome and food intolerance using low-GL principles.

Nigel works extensively with the media, with regular columns in the *Sunday Telegraph*, *Somerfield*, *Zest* and

Essentials magazines. His radio and television work includes BBC and ITN news programmes, Channel 4's *Fit Farm*, BBC's *Breakfast* and *Real Story*.

Nigel's first book, *The GL Diet*, was published in 2005, soon becoming a bestseller. His second book, *Nutrition for Dummies*, was published in autumn 2005.

Introduction: The Ultimate Diet

In my role as both a clinical dietician working on the front line with patients, and as a dietician working in the media, the question I'm asked most frequently has to be: 'What is the ultimate diet?'

It's a claim that's been made about so many of the diets that we now know to be at best useless and at worst dangerous. Before we can even begin to answer the question, I think we have to decide what the ultimate diet would need to include.

The ultimate diet – it works, it's easy to follow, it's based on sound scientific evidence, and it suits both men and women. There is no need to count points or calories or to weigh food. There is no humiliation or guilt! It is a diet for life – not just post-Christmas, and it's safe. There is such a diet and it's called the 7-day GL diet.

We know that every fad diet and every celebrity diet has maybe one or two of these attributes – but for me that's not good enough. For any diet to bear my name, and more importantly for me to use with patients in clinics, I have to be completely satisfied that my criteria have been met.

I firmly believe that if we don't have these high standards we will keep people in the 'diet trap', an unhealthy cycle leading to both physiological and psychological damage.

For me, the 7-day GL diet ticks all of the boxes. This isn't a diet we thought up sitting in our office – it's taken years of trials, research and adaptation to develop into a plan we are proud of and in which we have complete confidence.

From working with both men and women with weight issues I have learnt that while people like to have clear and simple guidelines, they are also more likely to succeed if given the responsibility of choice. This book will enable you to understand fully why the plan can work for you, and will help you to control your weight forever. What we want is for you to get to the point where you have learned enough to put the book away and get on with your life, without having to keep checking if you are doing things right.

The 7-day GL diet gives you the simple, flexible, straightforward foundations you need to start a new healthy way of eating. It will put you firmly in the 'weight-control driving seat' and keep you there!

Although it might seem like it, none of us goes upstairs one night thin and comes down the next morning with a weight problem – it takes years of repeated behaviour, and that behaviour becomes more ingrained with every failed dieting attempt. Writing the book has been both a professional and personal learning curve for all of us. Much of the advice, support and coaching we give to change these behaviours comes from our experience of working with real people, as well as from our personal stories of breaking free from our own 'diet traps'.

With a combined 90 years of dieting experience between us, we created Diet Freedom to help other people just like us, people with busy, pressured lives who were frustrated with the continual cycle of either preparing for the next diet, or recovering from the most recent dieting failure. Along with our individual professional strengths – tireless researcher, amazingly experimental cook and diligent dietician – this experience puts us in a unique position to support you in your own quest for diet freedom.

You may notice throughout the book references to both our website www.dietfreedom.co.uk and Diet Freedom Fighters. The name 'Diet Freedom Fighters' was coined by GL dieters on our website forums, who have taken up the GL challenge and are getting great results. We set up the website as an added support network and are delighted that it is so popular, not to mention huge fun. We love it and wanted to make sure you are aware that there is a lot more support available to you after reading the book – in fact, there's a whole community out there waiting to welcome you!

We really hope this book will give you the answers you have been looking for. We'd like to be the first to congratulate you on taking your first step towards success and achieving your goals!

Nigel Denby
Registered Dietician
RD BSc Hons

PART I

WHAT IS GL?

This section gives you all the background information about the diet and how it works. Most importantly, it tells you how to get started. It also explains why we feel the Glycaemic Load (GL) makes more sense than the Glycaemic Index (GI) alone, and gives you the simple science behind balancing blood sugars and permanent weight control.

You'll find:

- A simple explanation of how the diet works
- A clear guide to getting started
- Tips on deciding what you want to achieve

" After I had my son I'd gained about 10lb, and in the first few months I was so busy getting used to being a mum I didn't really have time to think about dieting. As the day to go back to work loomed closer and closer I began to panic. I'd got into a snacking habit that I just couldn't seem to break. I'd worked with Nigel on nutrition stories before, and after he talked me through the diet I quickly got back in control of my eating, and lost the weight I'd gained in time for my first day back at work. I felt so reassured that I hadn't needed to rely on a quick-fix diet. The concept of GL makes complete sense to me and has just become a way of life. "

Mishal Husain, BBC news anchor

Chapter 1

GI AND GL MADE SIMPLE

The first thing you probably want to know about this diet is: 'Does it work?'

Well, from my experience as a dietician working with patients in my own clinics, I can tell you yes, it most certainly does. Every day I see more and more people who previously thought they were stuck in a 'diet trap' telling me that the GL diet is finally getting them back in the driving seat where their weight is concerned. They are looking at life with renewed optimism and excitement as a world of possibilities and freedom opens up to them with every positive step they take towards their weight-loss goals.

Slow Carbs not No Carbs

Before we start looking at GI and GL and the differences in more detail, we need to go back a little further so you can see how our understanding of carbohydrate management has evolved.

A few years ago I was actively and publicly criticizing the 'high-protein, low-carb' diet phenomenon that was sweeping the world. We knew people were losing weight, but as a responsible dietician I could never sit comfortably with the idea of cutting out a whole food group from our diet.

What we can say about high-protein, low-carb diets today is this: in controlled weight-loss studies, they perform no better than any other weight-loss programme in the long term, and worryingly we remain unsure about how safe these diets are in terms of heart health and long-term kidney function.

So, let's get one thing straight: this is not a no-carb diet. The principle behind the GL diet is SLOW CARBS, and there's a big difference in terms of success and long-term health.

Although research into the Glycaemic Index (GI) has been carried out progressively over the last 20 or so years in Australia (University of Sydney) and Canada (University of Toronto), and more recently in the United States by Harvard Medical School,* the GI only really began to hit the headlines a couple of years ago as a possible, healthier successor to low-carb diets.

* The Harvard Medical School has carried out the longest running studies into human nutrition, stretching back over 20 years, and these are still continuing today.

How Can the GI Help Weight Control?

Foods that contain carbohydrates have an effect on our blood glucose (or blood sugars). This effect is measured as the 'glycaemic response'. A food that will make our blood glucose level rise quickly is classed as high glycaemic, whereas a food that has little or no impact on our blood glucose is low glycaemic.

When we eat high-glycaemic carbohydrates we get a rapid rise in blood glucose or a 'spike'. This is bad news for the body and prompts our pancreas to produce insulin, the most powerful hormone in the body, so not to be underestimated. Insulin comes rushing in to flush the glucose from our bloodstream as a safety mechanism and carries it to our liver and muscles, where it is stored as energy for later use. Healthy blood glucose is quite finely balanced – when blood glucose goes too low or too high it can detrimentally affect most of the organs in the body. If this situation becomes the norm it can have quite serious long-term health implications. The muscles and liver fill up very quickly, especially if we are not doing a lot of exercise to use up this 'stored energy' – by 'a lot' we mean the sort of training you might do to run a marathon. When the muscles and liver are full and can't store any more glucose, the only thing insulin can do is transfer the excess to other body tissues, where this excess energy is stored as FAT. Yes, those awful wobbly bits!

Once insulin has done its job and dispersed the glucose from our blood, the 'spike' in blood glucose falls rapidly. This is a vicious cycle as the rapid fall prompts us

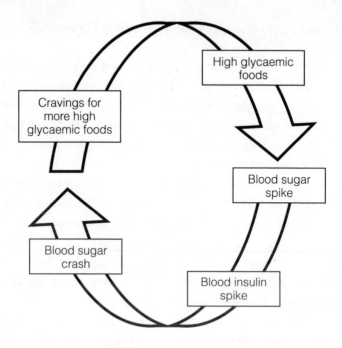

to crave more high-glycaemic foods – which actually caused the problem in the first place!

If we eat low-glycaemic foods, we store less excess energy and blood glucose levels are kept stable. This gives a slow-release, prolonged energy supply, enabling us to go about our activities with fewer cravings, feeling more balanced and ultimately storing less fat.

That's the basis of all low-glycaemic diets. But why low GL (Glycaemic Load) rather than low GI (Glycaemic Index)?

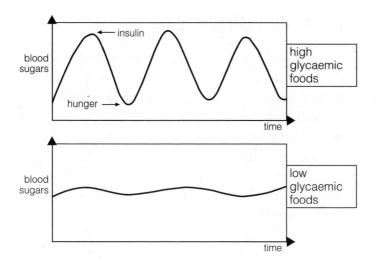

So What's Wrong with GI?

In principle nothing, except …

- The way the GI of a food is worked out doesn't always relate to the amount of food we actually eat at one sitting.
- GI can be very confusing.
- If you base your diet on low-GI foods, some very healthy foods are excluded, such as carrots, watermelon, parsnips, pumpkin and broad beans to name a few.
- GI gives us the first part of the story. It tells us that not all carbohydrates are equal. But that's a bit like knowing that you spend more money than you earn each month – it doesn't actually help you manage your money and get back in the black!

What's So Right about GL?

The Glycaemic Load (GL) gives you the whole story:

- GL allows you to understand with confidence how foods will affect your body.
- GL is based on carbohydrates in the portion sizes we usually eat, rather than the amount needed in a laboratory setting to work out the GI.
- GL means far more food choices.
- GL makes practical sense of the GI science. It's the final chapter in carbohydrate management and offers a real solution to long-term weight control.

The Technical Bit – How We Work out the GI and GL of a Food

Note: if you don't want to know about the science –
and you don't need to in order to follow the GL diet –
then skip to Chapter 2.

GI – the First Part of the Story

To work out the GI of a food, scientists take whatever amount of a food is needed to give you 50g of carbohydrate. Now, with a food like bread that isn't a problem because two slices of bread give us about 50g of carbohydrate. The bread is then fed to human volunteers and blood samples are taken from them at regular intervals to see how much glucose has been released into their bloodstream. The result of these tests is a GI number between 1 and 100.

Foods are classed as:
55 or less = low GI
56–69 = moderate GI
70 plus = high GI

So far, so good.

But let's look at another food. Take carrots and use the same procedure. To get 50g of carbohydrate from carrots you would need to consume about one-and-a-half pounds (0.7kg). That's a normal portion for a donkey maybe, but a bit excessive for the likes of us humans in one sitting. The volunteers (poor things) are fed the carrots, and the same blood tests and calculations are carried out as with the bread. The result is that carrots get a GI of about 75, making them high GI, which is why many GI diet books advise you not to eat them! Carrots are, in fact, a very healthy and low-'GL' food based on an average portion, so we can all thankfully continue to enjoy them as part of a balanced diet.

The GL Makes Sense of the GI

The GL goes a practical stage further. It takes the GI rating we've just outlined, but then very cleverly (thanks to Professor Walter Willett of Harvard Medical School who came up with the equation) takes into account the amount of carbohydrate in a portion of food we would normally eat. So now we know the effect a normal portion of carrots (around 100g) would have on our blood glucose levels, and that's what gives us the GL rating.

It's so simple and, more importantly, relevant to what we actually eat!

Foods rated using the GL do still get a number:

10 and under = low GL

11–19 = medium GL

20 plus = high GL

If you did want to count your GLs for the first few days to gain confidence that you are on the right track, you would be aiming to have 80GL or under on a low-GL day. A high-GL day would be 120GL or over.

BUT don't worry. Although we do give some basic portion guidelines and GL references, you don't have to count at all! Counting points and rigidly measuring and weighing foods is what turns us all off when it comes to diets. It's the bit that makes diets boring, boring, boring and, besides, who has the time?

All you need to do is read through the rest of the book, start loving healthy, low-GL foods, losing weight and, best of all, be able to keep it off forever as the GL diet becomes a way of life.

As serial dieters we are all searching for our own elusive 'diet freedom'. The GL finally brings this within everyone's grasp without deprivation or hunger.

For us, this GL plan is the ultimate permanent weight-loss solution because:

- It works – you'll see results in just seven days.
- It's easy to follow.
- It's based on sound, sensible science.
- It suits both men and women.
- There's no counting points.
- There's no endless weighing and measuring.
- There's no hunger or feeling deprived.
- There's no humiliation or guilt.
- It's a healthy diet you'll want to adopt for life, not just for Christmas …
- Oh … and it's safe!

Chapter 2

HOW TO FOLLOW THE 7-DAY GL DIET

OK, so now you've got the gist of how and why the GL diet works, are you ready to get cracking?

This chapter is designed to give you a short and sweet, whistle-stop tour of how to use the book, eat fantastic low-GL food from the 7-day plans and, of course, get results.

We have written *The 7-Day GL Diet* to give you enough guidance to guarantee results. You can start by making small changes a week at a time until, before you know it, you are actually living a healthy low-GL lifestyle. If all you want to do is follow the diet for seven days to lose a few pounds then that's no problem, but we'd like to think you'll want to carry on once we get you feeling all the benefits of eating low GL. Once you feel confident about which foods are low GL and which aren't, we think you'll want to join the thousands of successful 'Diet Freedom Fighters' (as they like to be known) out there who now make eating low GL part of their day-to-day routine. You can of course carry on using all the recipes, food lists and shopping guides long after the first seven days. Remember, this doesn't have to be a short-term quick fix – it can be a way of life.

Because the three of us are so different – and the feedback we've had tells us you are all so different too – we've carefully designed three seven-day plans to suit the variations in the way we all eat and prepare our food. If you want to pick one of the plans and follow it to the letter for seven days, that's fine; or if you prefer to mix and match, choosing meals from all of the plans, then that will work too. You can also follow each of the plans in succession for three weeks, checking your results as you go – do whatever is going to fit in with your lifestyle and feels right for you.

Whichever way you choose to use the plans, here are a few golden rules that will help you stay on track, and lose those unwanted pounds and inches.

The 7-day GL Diet Secrets of Success

- Whichever plan you want to follow, make sure you **eat three meals and two snacks each day.** This will prevent the dreaded hunger pangs you so often get on a diet, whilst ensuring you meet your nutritional needs for the day.
- **Use the shopping guides and food lists we have put together for you.** They are there to make everything easier and to ensure you don't find yourself at the supermarket checkout with a whole load of high-GL foods.

- **Get organized** – decide which day you want to start the plan, and stick to it. Get everything you need for at least the first two to three days. If you can, get rid of high-GL foods like biscuits, sweets, white breads and cakes that may act as trigger foods for you to fall off track.

- **Take some measurements** such as waist and hips as well as weight or BMI (body mass index – there is a BMI chart on our website) before you start and don't measure again until the end of the seven days. Weight can fluctuate daily for lots of reasons so you won't get a true picture of your success by jumping on the scales every day – and anyway, that's what people stuck in a diet trap do and you are now breaking free from all that!

- Although we have given some general guides for portions, **don't start weighing everything you eat!** There's no need. The guides are there just to give you an idea of a sensible portion. Maybe weigh a food once, and then you'll recognize the right portion the next time. **Do use the cupped hands portion guide** (see page 191) – this is the only portion rule you'll ever need!

- **Don't get hung up about counting GL points either.** Although we have given you the GL values of foods it's just to give you a basic understanding. We are all for 'Diet Freedom' and making everything smooth and easy, which fits in perfectly with this way of eating. Counting points and weighing food is too much like dieting for us – and remember WE HATE DIETS!

■ **Get active.** You will lose weight following the 7-day GL
   diet on its own, but this book is all about helping you
   towards a healthier lifestyle and that means moving
   about more (see page 18 for details). You will feel even
   better and get fantastic results if you increase your
   activity levels by even 30 minutes a day, along with
   following the eating plans.

So What Can You Expect from the 7-Day GL Diet?

A lot will depend on where you are starting from, what
your diet is like right now, how much you weigh, how active
you are, and of course how closely you follow the plans!

The one thing we can promise you is that you will lose
weight following the 7-day GL plan. You can expect to lose
between 2lb and 5lb in the first week, more if you've got a
lot of weight to lose. Unlike other diets, the difference is
that if you keep to a reasonably low-GL diet you'll keep
the weight off. If you just want to lose a few pounds then a
week or two following the plan may be all you need.
However, most people feel so well on the plans that they
carry on just for the many health and emotional benefits
(see research in Chapter 13).

For those of you who have more weight to lose it will
take a little longer, but you will get there, just take it seven
days at a time. Whatever your goals, we – and the many
wonderful Diet Freedom Fighters – are here to help and

support you. Check out our website to help keep you going.

You can use the plans for as long as you like. They are nutritionally balanced; there are no food groups you have to avoid; and above all you won't be hungry. Once you have got the hang of things it becomes second nature, but to start with we really recommend you take it in seven-day steps, building on your success as each week passes.

When you reach your goal we've also given you lots more help to maintain it (see Chapter 4).

The Seven-day Plans

Each of the 7-day plans has a particular type of person in mind. However, because we are complicated souls, and our daily routines aren't all the same, please remember you can jump into one plan today and another tomorrow. As long as you stick to a breakfast, lunch and evening meal plus two snacks from any of the plans you'll be just fine.

The Seven-day Fast and Friendly Plan

This is for people who probably know there is a cooker in the kitchen somewhere but don't have what you'd call a loving relationship with it. It's all about fast, healthy and delicious food to help you lose weight and snacks you can munch on the run. We even give you tips for eating out and grabbing ready prepared food.

The throw-together evening meals take no more than 20 minutes from start to finish, but if there's the odd night you do want to spend a bit longer cooking, no problem – just choose a recipe from the Foodie Friendly plan for keen cooks. Similarly, if you like to eat meat-free every now and then you can dip into the seven-day plan for vegetarians too.

What we wanted to give you was a fast, easy and convenient plan that fits in with your normal routine. This is Tina's speciality area – she's a great cook but far too busy to waste a minute more than she needs to in the kitchen.

Fast and GL-friendly is Tina's mantra!

The Seven-day Veggie Friendly Plan

This pretty much does what it says! Vegetarians are so often forgotten about when it comes to weight-loss plans, but not here. We have a mixture of quick, tasty recipes and one or two that take a little more time. The most important thing is that they taste fantastic – no more 'vegetarian lasagne' every night for you. Our recipes use clever ingredients, imagination and lots of variety to keep you nutritionally balanced and happy with fabulously indulgent food that's good for you and your waistline.

The Seven-day Foodie Friendly Plan

This is for the keen cooks amongst us. Deborah is a fantastically experimental cook who thinks nothing of starting preparation for a dinner party three days before anyone arrives – she's our domestic GL goddess.

Although you might not have quite as much passion as Deborah for cooking, this plan was designed for people who enjoy winding down at the end of the day by taking a little time to prepare dinner. The recipes aren't complicated but don't rely on convenience and time-saving tips. While they are all delicious, don't be fooled into thinking they must also be full of calories and luxury ingredients. We've kept a beady eye on our Deborah and have made sure these recipes will achieve the same weight-loss results as the other two plans.

Just in case you are wondering, I fall somewhere between Tina and Deborah when it comes to being bothered to cook – and would be the perfect example of someone who would mix and match from one plan to another throughout the week.

Activities!

OK, you know which plan you want to follow, or how you are going to combine the plans to suit your routine, so what else do you need? Ah yes, an activity plan. Don't panic – this is going to be so easy but we do think it's a really important part of your success.

If we asked whether you were prepared to find 30 minutes a day to get to your goals, what would you say? Just 30 minutes or 1800 seconds every day will do so much to move you towards your goals:

■ It will encourage your body to make new lean muscle tissue – that means your metabolic rate will speed up and you'll burn more calories even when you are asleep.
■ It will exercise your heart muscle and improve your overall health and wellbeing.
■ It will help you tone up as well as lose fat.
■ It will improve your quality of sleep.
■ It will help relieve stress and tension.
■ It will improve your overall physical and emotional fitness.
■ It will increase your results and make them even easier to maintain.

Every Second Counts! The 1800-second Challenge

Here's the challenge to get you moving about more and shedding those excess pounds. All we want you to do over the next seven days is find either one block of 30 minutes (1800 seconds), two blocks of 15 minutes (900 seconds) or three blocks of 10 minutes (600 seconds), and when you've got them we want you to walk for Diet Freedom. That's it! It's as simple as that – chuck on your trainers and start walking. Every step you take will lead towards your own personal Diet Freedom, and you will start to feel the benefits we've talked about very quickly. Your body will soon notice you're asking it to do more than usual if you are doing this every day, and that's when the changes will start to happen.

We find the best way to fit in those 30 minutes is to look at your routine and see where you could walk instead of drive or take the bus, or just take some of the time wasted sitting down watching television when you could be out and about.

Could you?

- Walk to work, or part of the way?
- Walk the kids to school?
- Cancel the papers and go and collect them yourself?
- Get out of the office at lunchtime?
- Take a walk when you get in from work?
- Get the kids away from the television or computer and walk with them?
- Walk the dog or someone else's dog?

The choices are endless. You might find it useful to have a couple of circuits in mind which will take you 10, 15 or 30 minutes, then you don't need to worry about where you are going to walk. Make sure you feel safe walking your circuits, and if you are worried about becoming more active check with your doctor first.

If you already go to the gym, take an exercise class, swim or whatever, that's great. But we want these 1800 seconds a day to be on top of what you already do.

Do this for the next seven days, then write a list of all the good things about getting more active – the pros. After that write another list of all the not-so-good things about getting more active – the cons. Which outweighs the other? We challenge you to come up with more cons than pros. If you do find some cons about your activity plan, look at each one in isolation and see if you can come up with a way to make it a good thing or a pro. Here's an example:

Pros and Cons of Getting Active for Seven Days

Pros	Cons	Solutions
Feel fitter	It's hard work	That's telling you how unfit you are – it will get easier and easier every day.
Losing weight	It's raining	That's life – buy a mac or an umbrella!
Losing inches	I feel silly	What's more silly – worrying about what other people think, or doing something really positive to change your life?

Pros	Cons	Solutions
Feel more toned	I haven't got time	What else takes you 1800 seconds? Ironing three shirts, cleaning the bathroom, watching a soap – think about your priorities.
Less breathless	I haven't lost a stone in a week	Good – that would be a crash diet and you'd almost certainly regain the weight. It took a long time to put the weight on, and it's going to take a while to lose it permanently.

More pros – can you think of any cons to match? – we couldn't!

Sleeping better		
Feel more confident		
Feel less stressed		
Feel kinda sexy!		
Clothes fit me		

Please add a few of yours too:

How Do I Know if I'm Walking Hard Enough?

That's an easy one. The 'talk test' is a really simple way of judging whether you are walking fast and hard enough. While you are walking, start talking (even to yourself!). Yes, people may stare but that's their problem. If you can talk away as normal you can probably go faster or include more of an incline on your circuit. If you can still talk but need to catch your breath you are spot on and can keep going. If you can't talk, have turned purple and keeled over, you are probably trying too hard.

Seriously, don't go mad. Start gradually and build up to a level that just gets you feeling a little warmer and increases your breathing rate. At some point that level will feel quite normal and will require little or no effort. That's the time to see if you can go faster, harder or longer.

So what's stopping you? Rise to the Diet Freedom walk challenge – we know you can do it!

Now you've got everything you need to get started: you know how the diet works, you know how to make the 7-day plans work for you a week at a time, and you're ready to start walking towards Diet Freedom – congratulations! Of course you have already taken the most positive step of all by starting to read this book – so well done!

We'd love to know how well you're doing, so please do log on to the forums on our website and let us know.

PART II

WHOSE SIDE ARE YOU ON?

There's a lot more to permanent weight control than just knowing what to eat. In this section we address getting your head in the right place to get started and KOKO – that's keeping on keeping on once you've reached your goals. We also challenge you to find 1800 seconds a day to change your life forever …

You'll find:

- How to prepare your mind for the 7-day GL diet
- How to set goals, achieve them and keep on keeping on
  – KOKO
- How to get active – don't panic! It's easy!

" Finding Nigel Denby's GL diet book in a tiny village bookstore was my happiest ever accident. At 55, I'd just started GI dieting after failing on two of the main 'group-attendance', point-counting UK diets. I wanted the dieting Holy Grail, enjoyable as well as easy to understand, without counting or crazy nutritional principles. In GL I found my freedom, as if a burden had fallen off my back.

Armed with Nigel's clear explanation of nutritional principles and a few recommended new habits, I took baby steps in healthy eating rather than dieting, helped by the recipes and by learning from experience. I started to lose weight gradually and feel much better. I found the message-board on the website very supportive. The research team were responsive to my queries and uncertainties, and the shared wisdom, support and experience of many ex-dieters, now Diet Freedom Fighters, was invaluable. To us, the future is GL – a healthy, enjoyable way of life and weight management, easily shared with family and friends – rather than glum solo dieting. "

Marie M from Cambridge

Chapter 3

IT'S ALL IN THE MIND

Why do diets fail? Well, we've all been there. We're all fired up and ready to go. It's Monday morning, another weekend of overindulgence behind us, and it's D-day – we're about to start the diet!

Later that week, or even that day, things start to get a bit dodgy. Perhaps work is stressful, the kids are playing up, you're tired, hungry, disorganized or a multitude of other reasons and it's all too easy to decide the diet is just too hard or too much hassle. It then slips by the wayside, leaving us feeling lousy, disappointed, guilty and like a failure.

This probably sounds familiar to many of us … and is exactly what we're talking about when we describe the 'diet trap': a cycle of preparing for a diet, starting a diet, stopping a diet and feeling guilty about it.

The problem is that we repeatedly just accept this cycle and put our failure down to things like:

■ I haven't got any willpower.
■ I haven't got time to fuss about with diet food.

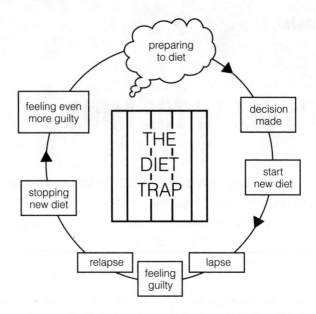

- I can only diet when everything is going smoothly in my life.
- I could diet if I lived on my own.
- I'll diet when things calm down at work.
- I'll diet when my social life quietens down a bit.
- Diets are really confusing – I just want something simple to follow.

Are these reasons or excuses for a diet failure? Well, they can be a bit of both, but what I see with so many of my patients, and from my own weight-loss experience, is that dieting behaviour is something we learn. The more times we go through that diet-trap cycle, the better we get at perfecting our destructive diet behaviour. Often the time it takes us to complete the cycle of starting the diet and feeling guilty about our failure gets shorter and shorter the more times we practise the cycle. In extreme cases this means that eventually some people don't even get as far as starting the diet – they believe they will fail before they start so what's the point in bothering at all?

All this can be changed. The diet-trap cycle can be broken right now, today, this second.

So, this is how to make the massive step out of your diet trap and turn your back on that miserable cycle forever ...

Remember: 'If you do what you always do, you'll get what you always got!'

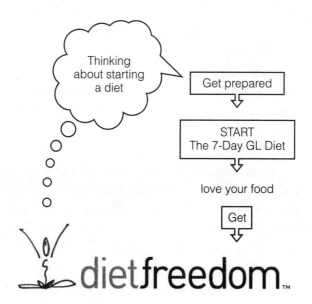

The first thing to do is accept that you have been stuck in a diet trap. If you're not sure, go back over the previous paragraphs and see if you recognize your own behaviour there.

If you already know this applies to you, think about the last time you started a diet-trap cycle and work through the list of questions below to help you unravel what really happened. For some of the questions I've given you answers some of my patients give me. Highlight the answer which best fits your story, or write in your own if none of them are appropriate, and then read on for some suggestions and tips on how to overcome and change your dieting behaviour.

What sort of diet did you choose?

A diet from a magazine
A diet a friend or colleague recommended
I just tried to cut down
I went to a slimming club
I always follow the same diet when I want to lose weight

Other _____

How did you plan for it?

I didn't

I told everyone I was on a diet and warned them not to tempt
me

I filled the fridge with diet food

I just played it by ear

I cancelled my social life

Other _____

What did you dislike about the diet?

The food was boring

I was hungry and just thought about food all day

The diet was really confusing so I had to guess what to eat a
lot of the time

It would have been fine if I was home all day, but eating out
was a nightmare

I ended up cooking different meals for the rest of the family

Other _____

What did you like about the diet?

I got results

It was really simple

I knew exactly what to eat and when

I was dieting with a friend and we kept each other going

My friends and family were really supportive

I had a clear goal to work towards

Other _____

What about eating out?

I'd starve all day so I could enjoy going out for dinner

I didn't eat out

Once I started eating out it was the slippery slope

I just ordered salads

Lunchtimes were the hardest; all I could get was a sandwich or
fast food

Other _____

Why did things start to go wrong?

I got really stressed and gave in to comfort eating

My weight loss slowed down and I got fed up

The effort just got too much for me

I had a lapse and just couldn't get back on track

Friends and family were trying to be helpful, but they were
driving me mad going on about my diet

Other _____

How did you feel when you realized you'd stopped dieting?

Relieved

Guilty

Angry and upset

It was inevitable

Hopeless

Other _____

OK, now you've got your answers in front of you, let's start to unravel them. Those answers are actually the most powerful tool you can use to help you break free from your diet trap. They are the roots of your diet behaviour and they open the door to breaking those behaviours and helping you start walking towards your own personal 'diet freedom'. Remember the phrase we used earlier?

> **'If you do what you always do, you'll get what you always got!'**

This is your chance to change this around to:

> **'If you change what you always do, you can get what you always wanted.'**

What Sort of GL Diet is Right for You?

The 7-day GL diet is designed to be very flexible. We've got plans for busy people who hate cooking, for vegetarians and for keen cooks. You just opt in and out of whichever plan suits you on each day; or if you know you're pretty consistent in your approach to food then pick a plan and follow it to the letter. We've always known that there is no universal diet which will suit everybody, but the science behind GL tells us that the principles of the diet can suit everyone. So we've taken those principles and made them work for everyone in a flexible format. If a friend has recommended the GL diet, you may need to approach it in a different way to them.

Our GL diet doesn't have a restrictive 'start-up' phase that leaves you feeling hungry, deprived and miserable. These plans have been designed to guarantee results. They are nutritionally balanced, so once you start you can just keep on going. We've also thought about eating on the run, and have given you comprehensive shopping and eating-out guides so you've got everything you need to make the GL choice a lifestyle in just seven days.

Planning for the 7-day GL Diet

Planning is vital. Think about the 4Ps:

Perfect
Planning
Produces
Permanent weight loss

You are about to change the way you eat, something you have done every single day of your life. If you just jump in without giving it a thought, isn't it likely you are going to make a mistake or forget something? Of course it is – one of the biggest causes of diet failure is that people don't plan enough.

By planning, we don't mean it needs to be a military exercise, but there are some basic requirements. You need to know what you are going to eat, the ingredients you require, and what you are going to do about food when you are away from home. The layout of the eating plans, recipes, shopping guides and food lists makes food planning as easy as possible. However, like any other tool, these are only helpful if you use them properly.

This is how we suggest you plan for your first week:

■ Take a quiet half hour or so the week before you want to start.
■ Sit down with the book and look at the eating plans.
■ Consult your diary and see what the week looks like. Will you be eating at home every night? Can you take your lunch with you to work? What about snacks? Do you need to remind yourself to take snacks out with you so you don't get caught out when you're on the hoof?
■ Choose a selection of meals and snacks from the plans which will fit in with your schedule, then look at the recipes and see what you'll need.
■ Write a list of everything you need – that's your personal weekly shopping list done.

You're off to the perfect start through perfect planning – easy!

After a week or two of doing this you'll get quicker and quicker at it, and it will begin to feel like second nature. Having everything you need at home is one of the most effective ways of successfully beating those old triggers to graze on sugary, fattening, high-GL snacks.

Making the 7-day GL Diet Work for You

Avoiding Boredom and Hunger Pangs

There is absolutely no reason for you to get bored or hungry on the diet. There are over 80 recipes to choose from. If you find yourself getting into a rut, go back to the recipes and find some new ones to add to your repertoire. If you are hungry then have another look at the plans and make sure you are following the guidelines and eating something every four hours. Snacking is an essential part of the GL diet. It's far better to pre-empt hunger than to wait until you are so hungry that you grab anything in sight! If you snack regularly and don't allow yourself to get too ravenous you are far more likely to choose something healthy.

Getting More Help and Advice

If there are specific foods or elements of the diet you are confused about, reread the book and check through the food lists and the 'Your Questions Answered' chapter to help give you the clarity you need. If you can't find the answers you are looking for in the book, do visit us online where you can get more help and support from us and from other Diet Freedom Fighters on the lively forums.

Eating Out

Don't panic if you've got a night out coming up. If you are eating out then find out what type of restaurant you'll be going to and use the eating-out guide to help you plan what you'll order. If you are just going out for drinks, then eat a sensible low-GL meal before you go and set a limit on the number of drinks you'll have during the evening.

Family Meals

Although you are following the GL diet to help you lose weight, there is no reason why the rest of the family can't eat low GL as well. Try not to get into the routine of cooking different meals for yourself. There's no need. You might want to give other members of the family a larger portion and not worry too much about how many potatoes or how much pasta you put on their plates.

Calling All Supporters

Before you start the diet, think about previous diets when you've been successful. Did you diet alone or with friends? A lot of people find it really helpful to 'buddy up' with someone, whereas others prefer to go it alone – there isn't a right or a wrong approach but it's well worth thinking about what will suit you best. Is there someone whom you think would be good to diet with? If you are going to diet with other people, choose carefully. There are diet saboteurs out there who can be really good at subconsciously spoiling your plan by encouraging you to take a shortcut here, or make a slip there. Make sure the person you choose is really committed and of a similar mindset to you.

Sometimes well-meaning friends and relatives just don't support us in the best way. Nagging, bullying and humiliating are thoroughly unhelpful, and guaranteed to make you stick two fingers up at the world and abandon your diet. Decide if you want to tell people you are trying to lose weight. If you do, decide what they can best do to help you and ask them for what you need. If you don't want them to eat biscuits in front of you, ask them not to. If you want them to ask how you are getting on once a week rather than every five minutes, or if you'd prefer them not to mention it at all, ask them. If you want them to query whether you should be eating certain foods, ask them to phrase the question in a way that doesn't sound accusing or patronizing. Decide on the kind of support you want and will respond best to and ask for it! If you prefer your support to come from people less involved with your day-to-day life then you can log on to our website and get an abundance of really helpful support.

A Word about Goal Setting

Take some measurements before you begin the diet so you can see how much weight you lose.

It's useful to know your BMI (body mass index). No weight-for-height charts are perfect but we prefer the BMI because it gives you an indication of the risk to your health from your weight. It's also useful because there is a wide range for each classification, and for people with a lot of weight to lose it's really helpful in setting staged targets. It's important to remember, though, that the BMI is a guide, not the Holy Grail.

For your reference there is a BMI chart on our website. There is good evidence that having a BMI of 20–22 has greater health benefits than a BMI of 23–25. However, we wouldn't recommend that you try to achieve a BMI of less than 18.5.

If your current BMI is between 20 and 25 then you really don't have a huge amount of weight to lose. You can probably expect a weekly weight loss of about 2lb as it tends to be slower the less you need to lose. If your BMI is between 25 and 30 you'll lose a little more each week, and if your BMI is above 30 then it wouldn't be unusual to lose more then 5lb in seven days, especially if you are able to be more active than usual, but check this first with your doctor.

It's also a good idea to take some body measurements such as your waist, hips and bust or chest. Use a tape measure and make sure you measure the same spot each time. Keep the tape measure straight for the most accurate result.

■ To measure your waist – measure around the naval or belly button
■ For hips – measure at the widest point of your bottom
■ For bust or chest – measure around your nipples

If you are working on increasing your day-to-day activity levels then measurements will be especially important. You may well change shape and lose inches faster than you lose weight. This is because as you increase your activity level, you replace some fat with muscle, which weighs more than fat. Physical measurements, especially around the waist, are just as meaningful as actual weight changes. Besides, if your goal is to drop a dress size or get into jeans two inches smaller than your current pair, does it really matter how much you weigh? No, of course it doesn't!

The more you move about, the less you'll wobble.

There's more information about goal setting coming up in the next chapter.

Chapter 4

KOKO – KEEP ON KEEPING ON

We talked in Chapter 3 about the importance of planning before you start your diet. Well, an integral part of the planning process is deciding what it is you actually want to achieve.

You might be thinking at this point: I'm reading a diet book, so I guess I just want to lose weight! I suspect that if we look a bit more closely at your motivations, we might find you've got quite a bit more to gain as well, and you can set goals for these outcomes too. You might want to feel more confident, be able to buy clothes more easily, lower your risk of heart disease, diabetes, cancer or other diseases, or improve your fitness. Of course your goal might be as simple as just wanting to get back into that dress or suit you haven't been able to wear for ages.

Whatever you want for yourself, the art of goal setting is keeping it real and achievable, and also having performance measures or milestones along the way to let you know you are heading in the right direction.

We've been very careful throughout the book to keep our promises real and achievable, and we really want to encourage you to do the same with your expectations of yourself. If you set unrealistic, unachievable goals for yourself you also set yourself up for disappointment and failure, and we all know what that feels like from our past experiences of diets, don't we?

Weight-loss Goals and Measuring Your Success

You may wish to find out your BMI (Body Mass Index) from the chart on our website. Remember, people with a BMI of between 20 and 25 should expect to lose no more than 2lb per week; people whose current BMI is between 25 and 30 could lose between 2 and 5lb per week; while people with a BMI higher than 30 may lose more than 5lb.

Weight loss is never consistent. No body loses the same amount of weight every week. So these guidelines are very much that – guidelines. A better way to look at weight loss, and the way I prefer to measure success with my patients, is to look at monthly weight loss. Taking three or four weight measurements during the month, and then averaging them over the full month, gives a much more accurate picture of what's going on. This method also evens out those weeks when weight loss is disappointing with those when you're walking on air because it's all going so well.

Each time you weigh yourself, it's important to use the same scales, and to weigh yourself at about the same time of day. This will prevent inaccuracies and also limit false weights from changes in fluid balance – we can weigh up to 4lb more at one end of the day just because we are holding more fluid – so same time, same equipment is a golden rule. When it comes to setting long-term targets for yourself, there are literally hundreds of options. We'll look here at a few of the most important.

Weight Loss for Health

If you are quite overweight – let's say your BMI is over 30 and you are dieting primarily for health reasons – then to set a goal of reaching a BMI of 20 might not be realistic. It may also be a goal that seems too far away right now, so it may not be that helpful in keeping you motivated. What might be more achievable would be to aim first of all to reduce your weight by 10 per cent. Let's say you currently weigh 16 stones (224lb or 101kg). A 10 per cent weight reduction would be $1\frac{1}{2}$ stones or 21lb or 10kg. The 10 per cent bit is very significant: good-quality studies have shown that reducing your weight by as little as 10 per cent significantly reduces your risk of heart disease, diabetes, high blood pressure, high cholesterol and some cancers – not to be sniffed at. Once you get to 10 per cent, aim for the next 10 per cent and so on. The health benefits just keep on coming.

Measurements

Measuring your waist, hips and bust or chest is another great way to chart your results. Fat carried around the tummy or abdomen is a key indicator for an increased risk of heart disease and diabetes. Aiming for a waist circumference that reduces your risk is a fantastic goal.

	Increased risk	Substantial risk
	Waist circumference:	*Waist circumference:*
Men	94cm (37 inches) or more	102cm (40 inches) or more
Women	80cm (32 inches) or more	88cm (35 inches) or more

We've also included a measurement chart for you to complete, below. This will be particularly useful if you think you'd like to continue the diet for a few weeks. It's a great motivator to let you know everything is moving in the right direction.

	Today	+4 wks	+4 wks	+4 wks	+4 wks	+4 wks	Target
Bust/chest							
Waist							
Hips							
Weight							
BMI							
Clothes size							

If you're not sure how to take accurate measurements then have a look at our tips on page 39.

Other Measures of Success

As far as other measures of success go, the key is to record where you are right now, before you even start the diet, and then make appointments with yourself to revisit your list and review your progress. You can do this for feelings, emotions, confidence and a whole host of weight-connected issues. There's much more to finding Diet Freedom than just what the scales tell you. You can score these feelings and emotions in a variety of ways. Words are good but if you find that difficult, try using the smiley face score or the scale of 1 to 10.

Smiley Face Score

 not very happy

 ok-ish

 still in hiding but feeling much better

 pretty darn chipper

 simply marvellous

Use the faces to represent how you feel for each feeling or emotion in the table below and watch your score get more and more smiley!

Scale of 1–10

Imagine a scale from 1 to 10, with 1 being the least confident or optimistic and 10 being the most confident or optimistic you could feel. Then give yourself a score for how you feel at that moment, and revisit the score table next week and the week after, and so on.

Scale of 1–10 for how you feel

1–2–3–4–5–6–7–8–9–10
1 = lowest
10 = highest

Keep a record of how you feel here:

	e.g.	Wk 1	Wk 2	Wk 3	Wk 4	Wk 5	Wk 6
Confidence	4 😟						
Optimism	9 😊						
Motivation	8 😃						
Fitness	3 😟						
Body shape	Tummy looks and feels flatter 😃						
Weight	11st 8lb						

Recording things other than your weight and physical measurements is a really motivating and important part of keeping you going. It might seem a bit strange to start with, but the more you do it, the easier it will become.

KOKO – Keep on Keeping on!

We'd love to take the credit for this phrase, but sadly we can't. It started with our army of Diet Freedom Fighters who keep each other motivated and share tips on our website forums. They are a great place to start when it comes to KOKO. Dieting can be a lonely old business and it's inevitable that you'll have good days and days when it all seems a bit too much. Those can be really negative and send your motivation into a downward spiral. Sometimes a trouble shared really can be a trouble halved, and you can bet that someone else is either feeling exactly the same as you, or has been there before and can give you just the words of wisdom and encouragement you need to get you back in positive mode. We regularly call in to the forums to update everyone with new information and encouragement, so please do join us and meet some new friends to share support and ideas with.

A Lapse is a Slip, a Relapse is a Return to Old Ways …

Lapsing, 'having a bad day', 'losing your focus' or 'falling off the wagon' – whatever you want to call it – is a perfectly normal part of changing. It's human nature to forget to have your morning snack occasionally, and end up choosing something unhelpful at lunchtime – that happens because you got too hungry to make a sensible choice, not because you have no willpower. Likewise, going to someone's house for dinner and eating a meal which doesn't quite fit in with low-GL principles is being polite, not weak willed. I have never worked with a patient who hasn't had the odd slip here or there, and I don't expect I ever will. If it were that easy to be perfect all of the time I doubt any of my patients would bother coming to see me, and you wouldn't have bothered to buy this book!

A lapse becomes a problem when it triggers all kinds of negative thinking, feelings of hopelessness, complacency and guilt:

- I've never had any willpower.
- I always give in to temptation.
- I've blown it.
- I'm miserable – let's eat – I'm even more miserable – let's eat some more …
- One biscuit won't hurt.

That's just the time when a lapse is in real danger of turning into a relapse, and within minutes you can be right at the end of that diet-trap cycle all over again. These are just the kinds of trick our negative dieting experience from the past likes to play on us. It's the way our old behaviour tries to exert power over the new relationship we have with food. The unhealthy food behaviours we have learnt, and relearnt, to perfection every time we have tried to diet in the past, enforce the negative self-belief thoughts like these promote. Part of finding your Diet Freedom is facing these thoughts head-on and beating them. A critical part of the process is seeing a lapse for what it is, understanding why it happened, deciding if you would deal with the situation differently in the future and moving on. End of story.

Temptation Tamers

One of the negative thoughts we've just talked about is the complacency thought – 'One biscuit won't hurt'. Well, no, in the grand scheme of things one biscuit won't mean you regain all the weight you've lost. It won't mean you suddenly increase your risk of heart disease or diabetes. One biscuit is not an international disaster! But, when you are trying to build a new relationship with food, one biscuit can lead to two, to three and to a whole packet. You can't remove all temptation from every aspect of life – Adam and Eve taught us that – but if you are aware that temptation will pass your door, you can be prepared.

Many of our Diet Freedom Fighters have told us that having some 'Temptation Tamers' ready for when the biscuits appear in the office or the pudding menu comes round at the restaurant are really helpful at making them stop, pause and make an informed choice about whether they want to give in to temptation or not. Have a look at this small selection. If any of them strike a chord with you, write them down and stick them on the fridge door, or put them in your purse or wallet – keep them somewhere handy for when temptation comes knocking.

- 'Just one will be the tip of the iceberg.'
- 'Bad for me, bad for my bum.'
- 'Junk-food junkie or health-food hero?'
- 'One small step for man, a giant step towards my Diet Freedom.'
- 'How long will that make me feel good for?'
- 'No thanks, that's what I used to do.'
- 'Junk food = lousy mood.'
- 'One biscuit is too many, a packet is never enough.'

Maintaining Your Weight

Eventually you will want to stop losing weight and focus on maintaining the great shape you're in. Because the GL diet is a way of life and not just a quick 'here today, gone tomorrow' fad, maintaining your weight doesn't mean you jump straight back into your old ways – that would just be an extended form of the diet-trap cycle and is definitely not a good move. The likelihood is that, by now, you'd actually find it very difficult to go back to those horrible crash-and-burn days of fluctuating blood sugars, mood swings, irritability and, of course, weight gain.

What you can do when you want to maintain your weight is relax a little more when you're eating out. You might choose to have a little more alcohol (and no, we don't mean binge drinking!) or to have the odd dessert, some extra bread or other moderate-GL foods.

The 80/20 Rule

Many people find the 80/20 rule a good way of keeping themselves on the right track during maintenance. The 80/20 rule is about choosing sensibly most of the time, and having a little of what you fancy some of the time. This guide often fits in to the working week, watching what you eat Monday to Friday and relaxing more at the weekend. Please, please, don't take this as the green light to go hell for leather at the weekend. It's a sad but true fact that everything we put in our mouths has an effect on our bodies, and we simply can't get away with bingeing and then starving ourselves to try and make up for it. That's bordering on an eating disorder and stands for everything we're against.

The 80/20 rule is fine when you feel very comfortable with your relationship with food, and when you are also really enjoying your GL lifestyle. If you don't feel safe letting your guard down, then don't do it yet. Wait a while and come back to it in a few weeks' time. Go at your own pace.

KOKA – Keep on Keeping Active

This is another important part of KOKO. As we've said before, you don't have to go exercise mad to be healthy and lose weight, but it really helps if you can be more active. Again, by now we'd hope that your daily 1800 seconds are no longer a chore and have become an invigorating part of your routine. If that's the case then congratulations – you are now a naturally active person and have significantly increased your chances of a longer, healthier life!

When it comes to maintaining your health and weight, your activity levels are just as vital as they were when you were losing weight. This might also be a good time to look at increasing your daily activity levels further, especially if you intend to try the 80/20 rule.

I often advise my patients to view their activity like a savings bank when they are in weight maintenance. If you put in regular deposits, you can make an occasional withdrawal and still stay in credit. This applies in exactly the same way to your energy balance – expend energy through activity every day, and every now and then you can have a little extra intake without piling on the pounds. Unlike your bank account, there is no overdraft limit when it comes to weight control, so don't be fooled into thinking that an extra circuit around the park once a week gives you enough credit to party all weekend and keep out of the red!

When maintaining your weight, the bottom line is:

- Use your common sense.
- Start gently with your maintenance plan, and find the level that suits your body.
- Remember, it takes a lot longer to burn off excess energy through activity than it does to consume excess energy through food and drink.

Chapter 5

EVERY SECOND COUNTS

In Chapter 2 we talked about increasing your activity through walking with the 1800-second challenge. Getting active is such an important part of a healthy weight-loss plan that we are going to get back on our soapbox again! As well as scheduling your eating plan, social life and support networks, this is also a good time to plan in that activity.

We've concentrated on walking because it's cheap and so easy to do, but there are lots of other activities which will get that heart muscle working and help you build that all-important lean muscle tissue. Remember, muscle tissue increases your metabolic rate and helps you burn more fat, even when you're asleep!

If walking doesn't float your boat then find something else that will get you moving:

- Dancing
- Cycling
- Swimming
- Fitness classes
- Roller-blading

- Trampolining
- Skipping
- Sex

These are all activities you can measure in terms of their frequency and duration – yes, the sex too! You're looking for that magic 1800 seconds or 30 minutes every day. Then you can rest on your laurels and feel 100-per-cent confident you are being active enough to:

- Lose weight faster and keep it off
- Boost your immunity
- Get a natural high from increased production of endorphins (feel-good hormones)
- Sleep better
- Boost your brain and memory power
- Reduce your risk of heart disease, diabetes, cancer and high blood pressure

And if all this still sounds just too much then start by focusing on your day-to-day routine, and work out where those 1800 seconds can be found in tasks you have to do anyway. Here are some ideas:

- Walking to and from work
- Walking the children to school
- Using the loo on another floor – take the stairs
- Going out to get your lunch – take a longer route
- Housework
- Cleaning windows

- Mowing the lawn
- Digging
- Washing the car
- Sex – not that sex should ever be routine of course!

Day-to-day tasks are so useful for building up your total activity level. It's just as effective to find your extra 1800 seconds in short bursts if one block of 30 minutes isn't practical or possible.

Exercise Options for Less Mobile People

If you are one of those people who, for whatever reason, are unable to get about as well as most of us, please don't take our emphasis on activity as meaning you won't get results on the 7-day GL diet. You will. It may mean it takes you a little longer to reach your goals but it is possible to achieve weight loss by changing your diet alone.

If walking is a real problem for you then chair exercises can be very helpful. Some people find that swimming can also be great because the water supports their weight rather than their joints having to do the work. It's really important to take advice from your health-care professionals before embarking on an activity plan. You may also find that your GP's surgery or physiotherapy department can offer advice and ideas for less able people to increase their activity levels. Above all, don't let your mobility difficulties prevent you from reaching your weight-loss goals.

" Having been on every diet written, I am always hoping for a miracle. I bought the GL book hoping this would be the one. At last I've found something realistic. The main reason is you really do have 'freedom' – no counting, no visits to supermarkets checking every packet for salt, fat, carb and calorie content. The book is easy; it all makes sense; the recipes are delicious and suitable for everyone; you don't need to sit eating differently from the rest of civilization.

I have now lost 10lb – it' not fast but it's constant. I feel healthier and have noticed how much more energetic I am. I'm also shrinking in different places! This message is from a real person. I'm not a stick insect – I'm still a larger-than-life lady – but for the first time in many years I now have real hope that this is going to work and become a way of life. "

Andie M from Essex

PART III

YOUR 7-DAY GL GUIDES

There's something for everyone in the 7-day GL diet plans: a plan for the fast and furious; a veggie-friendly plan; and one for adventurous, keen cooks. You can choose one plan that suits you, or mix and match. The beauty of the 7-day GL diet is its flexibility.

In this part of the book, you'll find:

- The 7-day Fast and Friendly Plan
- The 7-day Veggie Friendly Plan
- The 7-day Foodie Friendly Plan
- Lots of extra recipes – even an amazing chocolate celebration cake!

Shopping lists for all three plans can be found in Chapter 11.

❝ I'm just delighted to let you know that it's exactly six months since I started my new low-GL lifestyle. My weight today is 14st 4lb. This is just over my halfway point as I have now lost 4st 4lb! I started at 18st 8lb so I have just under 4st to go. On average, I have lost 2lb per week, with some weeks as much as 3lb. Others, like my 60th birthday week, I lost nothing but didn't gain, despite a whole weekend of partying! I am also pleased that I've been able to cut down the number of tablets I take. Prior to GL, I was taking 14 tablets every day for various chronic conditions. Now I am on just two tablets for blood pressure.* I'm off to the doctor this week to see if I can knock one of these off too. ❞

Pauline H from Kirkham, Preston

* Always take advice from your doctor before altering any medication.

Chapter 6

THE 7-DAY FAST AND FRIENDLY PLAN

OK, so you have landed on this page because you are short of time, and have no enthusiasm whatsoever for getting the oven gloves out. Am I right? Well, I'm with you there … who can be bothered? I do love good food, and it *has* to taste fantastic, but I have little time for anything other than making it look attractive, admiring it briefly and then eating it. I greatly admire Deborah's stove method and marinating techniques (see Chapter 8), but for me … well, the fact is that I don't really want to look at food ingredients or mess around with them for any longer than I absolutely have to. Call it a low boredom threshold or an oven allergy but I'm sure I can't be the only one!?

So, don't worry. You won't need to peel or scrape anything, remove the million layers of a garlic clove thingy or attempt to de-knobble a piece of ginger whilst trying to keep your fingers intact. Oh no, if it can't be rustled up in a nanosecond I'm out of the kitchen and back at the computer. So in order to eat good, healthy food that can be prepared in a flash I am always looking for healthy shortcuts to scrumptious low-GL meals and snacks.

We all have our own reasons for wanting food that is quick to prepare but still delicious and healthy.

For busy execs racing around town with hardly a second to themselves, healthy grab-and-run, quick-to-prepare food is a necessity – either that or starve.

Then there are those of us who work nine-to-five. We grab breakfast as we go out the door – if we're lucky – and then have to endure the perils of the staff canteen. The less said about that the better! Is your staff canteen a place you fear to tread, particularly when hungry and doing your darndest to lose weight? You might start the day with good intentions. Perhaps you will have a prawn salad for lunch. But then the stress of the day takes over, and the lure of fish and chips or stodgy lasagne gets the better of you.

Well, fear not. Eating low-GL helps knock out the nasty cravings. You will feel incredibly virtuous when whipping out your tempting low-GL lunch box or portable feast that you can throw in the communal microwave at work.

Last, but by no means least, the Fast and Friendly Plan is ideal for busy mums and dads. They are often juggling so many balls in the air that they don't realize they aren't eating the best diet for busy folk.

Feel free to mix and match between the three diet plans. We hate dieting and, most of all, prescriptive formats that get you all worked up and anxious over every scrap of food you consume. Deep contemplation about whether you have strayed a couple of points over your starvation level limit for the day is now firmly consigned to the bad old days. No, you don't have to go to bed at 6pm to ensure you don't go near the fridge again and be tempted to go over your points limit for the day!

For a shopping list for this plan, please see Chapter 11 (pages 218–22).

You will find 'guide' lines here but no rigid rules – hurray! So, let's get started …

Where oatcakes, crispbreads or slices of bread are mentioned in the plan, men should have up to 4 oatcakes/crispbreads or 2 slices of bread; women should have up to 2 oatcakes/crispbreads or 1 slice of bread.

Eating regularly – every four hours – is important to help balance your blood sugar levels so try not to skip meals and snacks.

	Day 1	Day 2	Day 3	Day 4	Day 5	Day 6	Day 7
Breakfast	Continental breakfast: 2 slices of ham (not plastic), 2 slices of cheese and sliced beefsteak tomato – bit of black pepper	2 boiled eggs, low-GL toasted bread with olive oil-based spread (see food list for recommended breads)	1 tbsp of plain, natural, sugar-free yoghurt, topped with strawberries and a small handful of pine nuts	Bran sticks (sugar free) from health-food store with milk or soya milk and a handful of chopped dried apricots thrown in	3 lean bacon rashers, 1 egg and 1 small tin of reduced-sugar beans	Chopped peach, apple and grapes in a bowl topped with a dollop of unsweetened plain Greek yoghurt	2 rye crispbreads topped with cottage cheese and sliced pear
Snack	25g dark chocolate (at least 70% cocoa)	Small handful of almonds	Small handful of sunflower seeds	Small pot of cottage cheese	Small handful of pine nuts	A couple of cheese sticks	Handful of grapes

	Day 1	Day 2	Day 3	Day 4	Day 5	Day 6	Day 7
Lunch	Asparagus soup	Microwaved sweet potato with cream cheese and side salad	Tomato and herb soup	Egg mayonnaise salad	2 rye crispbreads topped with houmous	Open sandwich with low-GL bread, layered with ham, salad and coleslaw	Prawn salad with coleslaw
Snack	Oatcake with cream cheese and tomato	A nectarine or peach	A rye crispbread with sugar-free peanut butter	Handful of cherries	An apple	Oatcake with olive-oil spread	25g dark chocolate (at least 70% cocoa)
Dinner	*Avocado and Prawns	*Spicy Chicken Salad with balsamic vinegar and olive oil	*Pan-fried Tuna Steaks with Tomato Sauce	*Fast Fettuccine Bolognese	*Greek Salad	*Pesto Salmon	Gammon steak with poached egg, peas and a mixed side salad

* Recipes for these dishes are given in the following pages.

Recipes for the Fast and Friendly Plan

The following recipes are designed for speed. You can use the microwave or, in most cases, pan-fry or bake in the oven if you prefer.

Avocado and Prawns

Preparation time: 5 minutes, Serves 2

2 large ripe avocados (if it's ripe it will feel slightly soft if you
    press the end gently)
2 large handfuls shelled prawns
2 tbsp mayonnaise
Squeeze of lemon juice (fresh or bottled)
1 tbsp tomato sauce or purée
Large pinch paprika (optional)
Large handful cashew nuts

Cut the avocados in half lengthways and carefully remove the stones. Fill each half generously with prawns. Combine the mayonnaise, lemon juice and tomato sauce to make a dressing and spoon over the prawns. Sprinkle paprika over the dressing. Scatter cashew nuts over the top. Serve with a large crunchy mixed salad.

Spicy Chicken Salad

Preparation time: 5 minutes, Cooking time: 2 minutes, Serves 2

1 cos lettuce, washed
2 tbsp sun-dried tomatoes (you can buy these in oil in
     tubs/jars – drain well and use as you need them) or
     8 cherry tomatoes, halved
½ large cucumber, peeled and sliced
1 small red onion, sliced thinly
1 tbsp balsamic vinegar
2 tbsp extra virgin olive oil
Large handful pine nuts
Freshly ground black pepper
8 small spicy precooked chicken fillets (you can buy these
     chilled with various flavourings from all supermarkets)
1 tbsp grated Parmesan cheese

Tear the lettuce into chunky pieces and put in a large bowl. Add the sun-dried or cherry tomatoes, cucumber and onion. Drizzle with the balsamic vinegar and olive oil, add the pine nuts, grind some black pepper over and toss to combine. Heat the chicken pieces in a microwaveable dish in the microwave for around 2 minutes or until heated through. Cut the chicken into smaller pieces and add to the salad. Combine and serve with a sprinkling of Parmesan cheese over the top.

Pan-fried Tuna Steaks with Tomato Sauce

Preparation time: 5 minutes, Cooking time: 2 minutes, Serves 2

½ tbsp extra virgin olive oil
2 fresh tuna steaks
Freshly ground black pepper
Squeeze of lemon juice
1 jar of tomato-based sauce (any pasta-type sauce will
    be fine)

Warm the oil in a deep frying pan and add the tuna steaks.
Grind black pepper over the top and add the lemon juice.
Cook each side for a couple of minutes until almost
cooked through. Pour over the jar of tomato-based sauce
and cover, heating gently until the tuna and sauce are
cooked through. Serve with a large tin of butter beans
(empty into a microwaveable dish and cook for about
2 minutes until heated through), and freshly cooked
broccoli.

Fast Fettuccine Bolognese

Preparation time: 10 minutes, Cooking time: 10 minutes, Serves 2

200g fettuccine or similar fresh egg-based pasta (you can use
   dried pasta or spaghetti)
200g/1½ cups lean minced beef
1 carton passata – about 500g (Italian sieved tomatoes,
   available from supermarkets)
Freshly ground black pepper
1 tbsp cream/crème fraîche (optional)
Cherry tomatoes, halved (to garnish)
1 tbsp Parmesan cheese

Cook the fettuccine lightly for a few minutes in a pan of
boiling water until *al dente*, or just cooked. Drain and set
aside. Place the mince in a large microwaveable bowl in the
microwave and pour over the passata. Grind over some
black pepper and stir. Cover and cook for about 4
minutes, stirring after each minute. Stir in the cream or
crème fraîche and cook for a further 30 seconds.

Place the fettuccine on a plate and spoon over the
mince and sauce mixture. Garnish with halved cherry
tomatoes around the plate and sprinkle Parmesan over
the top.

Greek Salad

Preparation time: 5 minutes, Serves 2

4 vine-ripened tomatoes, quartered
1 small red onion, sliced thinly
½ large cucumber, peeled and sliced
100g/½ cup feta cheese, cubed
100g/½ cup black olives
2 tbsp wine vinegar
3 tbsp extra virgin olive oil
Freshly ground black pepper

Mix the tomatoes, onion, cucumber, feta cheese and olives in a bowl. Pour over the vinegar and oil, season with black pepper to taste and serve.

Pesto Salmon

Preparation time: 5 minutes, Cooking time: 2 minutes, Serves 2

2 boneless salmon fillets (fresh or frozen)
1 tbsp pesto (jars available from supermarkets) – any type
Squeeze of lemon juice

Place the salmon fillets in a microwaveable dish with 2 teaspoons of water. Spread the pesto evenly over the top of each fillet and squeeze lemon juice over the top. Cover and cook for 2 minutes in the microwave or until cooked through. Alternatively, bake in a moderate oven in the same way in an ovenproof dish – cover with foil and cook for 10 minutes or until cooked through.

Serve with 3 or 4 new potatoes or a baked sweet potato and peas.

Lunch Box Ideas

- Rye crispbreads, oatcakes, any of the low-GL breads from the food list or a wholemeal pitta are good bases.
- Olive oil-based spread is a good choice as it contains no trans/hydrogenated fats.
- A pot of cottage cheese, cheese sticks, cream cheese triangles and mini Edams are great and very portable.
- You can buy great mixed bean pots from supermarkets now, often in a vinaigrette – fast, friendly and full of fibre!
- Pots of smoked salmon, crab, mackerel or other fish-based pâtés are healthy, quick and easy choices.
- You can buy various natural dips and spreads from supermarkets – cheese and chive, garlic and herb, sour cream and chive, salsa and houmous are just a few that are widely available and make good lunch-box fare.
- Add some carrot sticks, celery sticks and sliced peppers and you have some good dippers.
- Take some fruit and chop it up at work, or chop and put it in a sealed container in the morning with some lemon juice over it to stop it browning.
- Wash some raspberries and strawberries and take to work to stir into a pot of Greek or bio yoghurt with a handful of pine nuts.
- Throw a handful of walnut pieces over a small tub of Greek yoghurt and dip in some fresh peach cut into quarters. Great for the lunch box or a grab-and-run snack.
- Half a melon or some watermelon slices wrapped in cling film would be a great lunch-box basic.

- Any small pots of sugar-free yoghurt can be used, or buy a big pot of plain yoghurt and decant different chopped and dried fruits into a smaller container to take to work each day.
- Boiled eggs travel well – take some mayonnaise sachets and a crunchy salad in a Tupperware box and mix when ready.
- Cold chicken, turkey, ham, pork and beef are great with salad – add some coleslaw and you have a filling lunch.
- If you have a microwave at work you can take a washed sweet potato, prick all over with a fork and cook for about 5 minutes until soft inside. Fill with sour cream, any kind of cheese and black pepper – delicious. Or why not take a carton of fresh soup? Or make your own soup in the blender at home and heat it up at work.

Snack Ideas

- A few squares of dark chocolate are a great standby snack.
- A handful of dried apricots, apple or any berries is also great – be careful with dried cranberries as they often have sugar added to them.
- A mini Edam or pot of cottage cheese
- An apple, pear, orange, handful of grapes, a nectarine or any of the low-GL fruits.
- A handful of any nuts (unsalted) makes a good snack but eat no more than a handful a day as they are very dense in calories.

- A small pot of sugar-free yoghurt will keep you going until the next meal. A couple of oatcakes or rye crispbreads with cottage cheese or peanut butter would do the same.

About Town

You can normally get something reasonably healthy and low GL now from most sandwich and coffee bars.

- Go for the mixed salads or filled pitta breads. Pots of four-bean salads in vinaigrette are also a good choice.
- Pots of chopped fruit are often available. You can even get filled fruit bags and a choice of salads from fast-food joints now!
- Pots of yoghurt are also becoming popular in coffee bars but they are often high in sugar – check the label.
- If you are eating out, stick with the most natural options available – a basic chicken or fish dish with salad or low-GL vegetables is always on offer. Don't worry if you have to ask the waiter to adapt the dish slightly – they are used to it!
- If you have a coffee make it a plain coffee or a cappuccino as many of the more adventurous sounding coffees in coffee bars contain glucose syrup.
- Many so-called natural energy bars are full of sugar and glucose syrups. Although you may get a quick energy fix, it will be followed by a crash and leave you feeling

tired and unenthusiastic about the rest of the day. A better choice would be a few squares of dark, cocoa-rich chocolate that has very little sugar and at least 70 per cent cocoa. You can buy this from all supermarkets now, and smaller bars are available in health-food shops.

" Having tried several diets that have either been a total failure or required a major lifestyle alteration, I'm thrilled with how I'm doing now. Since finding the GL diet I have lost 2st 4lb in just nine months. It fits with my lifestyle and I certainly have more energy. **"**

Caroline E from East London

Chapter 7

THE 7-DAY VEGGIE FRIENDLY PLAN

This plan, for the veggies amongst us, falls somewhere between the 'Fast and Friendly' and the 'Foodie Friendly' plans in terms of time spent in the kitchen. There are shortcuts aplenty that you can take too.

For example, if mashing avocados or chickpeas is not your thing, you can find perfectly acceptable guacamole and houmous in most supermarkets. If you prefer to make your own, there is a great recipe for both of these in the 'Foodie Friendly' plan. A whole range of salads in pots are also readily available in the shops and needn't be handmade, so don't let the fact that there are recipes for bean and lentil salads bring you out in a sweat! Nut burgers and unsweetened yoghurts ditto.

We've included muesli in the breakfast choices – you can either buy one of the unsweetened versions or you'll find a recipe for Diet Freedom Muesli on page 112.

Lots of fresh herbs and garlic are included in the recipes. These give a great boost to the flavour and aroma of the finished dish, but don't be afraid to use dried herbs – you will still get a good result. You can freeze fresh herbs once washed as they wilt very quickly. There's quite a bit of garlic in this plan (and the Foodie Friendly one). It's really good for you, but if you don't like it, or any of the other herbs and spices, just leave them out.

In Chapter 8 we have included lots more delicious veggie recipes, including some great veggie side dishes, salads and mash. There are also some really lovely dressings, snack alternatives and even one or two desserts. Please feel free to mix and match – we want everyone to love their food as well as their body!

For a shopping list for this plan, please see Chapter 11 (pages 223–8).

Where oatcakes/crispbreads or slices of bread are mentioned in the plan, men should have up to 4 oatcakes/crispbreads or 2 slices of bread; women should have up to 2 oatcakes/crispbreads or 1 slice of bread.

Eating regularly – every four hours – is important to help balance your blood sugar levels so try not to skip meals and snacks.

	Day 1	Day 2	Day 3	Day 4	Day 5	Day 6	Day 7
Breakfast	*Porridge	Scrambled eggs with fresh herbs on low-GL toast	Fresh low-GL fruit with Greek yoghurt	Low-GL toast with Marmite and cheese	Grilled tomatoes on low-GL toast	Muesli (with no added sugar)	Quorn sausages, grilled tomatoes and reduced-sugar baked beans
Snack	Handful of dried apricots	Oatcakes with guacamole	Small pot of *Lentil and Tomato Salad	Small pot of natural yoghurt with honey and toasted seeds	Small *Bean Sprout Salad with houmous	*Avocado and Tomato Pot	Small handful of brazil nuts
Lunch	*Salad 'Bisbas' with houmous and oatcakes	*Spicy Bulgur Wheat and Butter Bean Salad	*Nutty Chickpea and Sesame Burgers with salad	*Curried Butternut Squash Soup	*Avocado, Tomato, Mozzarella and Spinach Salad	*Mushrooms on Low-GL Toast	*Butter Bean and Avocado Salad with *Heavenly Grilled Pepper Dressing

	Day 1	Day 2	Day 3	Day 4	Day 5	Day 6	Day 7
Snack	Small pot of *Bean Salad	Sliced pear with piece of cheddar	Avocado with fresh lemon juice and toasted seeds	Apple and cheese stick	1 small pot *'Lemon Heaven'	Oatcakes with no-added-sugar peanut butter	Houmous with crudités
Dinner	*Baked Sweet Potato with Cheese and Tomato	*Nutty Chickpea and Sesame Burgers with low-GL veggies	*Zesty Vegetable Kebabs with Wild Rice and Chickpeas	*Asparagus, Lemon and Mint 'Barleyotto'	*Toasted Courgette, Garlic and Basil Pasta	*Vegetables 'Greek Style' with chickpeas and wild rice	*Tomato and Cauli Crumble with greens

* Recipes for these dishes are given in the following pages.

Recipes

Porridge

Preparation time: 2 minutes, Cooking time: 5–10 minutes, Serves 1

225g/1 cup old-fashioned porridge oats
500ml/2 cups water
1–2 tsp fructose or 1 tsp honey
1 tbsp natural yoghurt, crème fraîche or cream

Put the oats and water into a microwaveable bowl and microwave until cooked. Or put in a small saucepan over a medium heat and stir until cooked. Stir in the fructose or honey at the end to taste. Put into a bowl, add a nice big dollop of natural yoghurt, and enjoy.

Optional Extras
- Stir in some frozen berries halfway through cooking.
- Add a chopped apple or pear, or some chopped dried apricots, at the end.
- Stir in some reduced-sugar jam.

Salad 'Bisbas'

Preparation time: 10 minutes, Serves 2 as a main course, 4 as a side salad

This is an adulteration of a Tunisian salad. Really different from the norm, it's delicious with houmous and low-GL bread or oatcakes.

150g/½ cup radishes, chopped into small pieces
4 tbsp parsley, chopped finely
2 fennel bulbs, washed and chopped into small pieces
1 packet rocket
Juice and rind of 1 fresh lemon
Freshly ground black pepper
2 tbsp extra virgin olive oil
200g/2 cups pitted olives (whichever type you prefer)

Mix all the ingredients together, dress with the olive oil and serve. If you are taking this in a box for lunch, keep the rocket separate and dress the rest of the salad so the flavours steep. Add the rocket and combine just before eating.

Bean Salad

Preparation time: 10 minutes, Serves 4 as a side salad

Choose any two from:
1 can (usually 410g)/2 cups chickpeas, drained and rinsed
1 can haricot beans, drained and rinsed
1 can kidney beans, drained and rinsed

1 spring onion, diced finely (optional)
4 sun-dried tomatoes, chopped finely
Generous handful of basil, chopped roughly
Freshly ground black pepper
Dash of Tabasco
1 tbsp balsamic vinegar
2 tbsp extra virgin olive oil (or oil from the sun-dried tomato
    jar)
Juice of ½ a lemon

Drain and rinse the beans, put into a bowl with all the
other ingredients, mix well and serve. Great as a side salad
or lunch pot.

Baked Sweet Potato with Cheese and Tomato

Preparation time: 10 minutes, Cooking time: 4 minutes or 40, Serves 1

1 small sweet potato
1 large tomato, chopped into small chunks
Small handful basil, torn
40g/½ cup grated Cheddar cheese
Freshly ground black pepper

Bake the sweet potato – for about 40 minutes in the oven, or until cooked in the microwave. Put the chopped tomato in a sieve over the sink to drain, then mix in a bowl with the basil (saving some to garnish). Slit open the cooked sweet potato and mash half the Cheddar cheese into the cooked flesh. Then top with the tomato mix, grind over lots of black pepper, sprinkle on the remaining cheese and top with the remaining basil.

Other Great Toppings
- Reduced-sugar baked beans
- Bolognese
- Tomato salsa
- Herby guacamole
- Houmous

Spicy Bulgur Wheat and Butter Bean Salad

Preparation time: 15 minutes, Cooking time: 10 minutes, Standing time: 1 hour, Serves: 2, or 4 as a side salad

2 tbsp extra virgin olive oil

1 red onion, diced

2 garlic cloves, grated or crushed

1 tsp ground cumin

350ml/1½ cups vegetable stock

120g/⅔ cup bulgur wheat

2 tomatoes, peeled and chopped

120g/⅔ cup butter beans, drained and rinsed

6 tbsp fresh parsley, chopped

6 tbsp fresh coriander (cilantro), chopped (optional)

6 tbsp fresh mint, chopped

1 fresh green chilli, seeded and finely chopped (or generous pinch powdered chilli, or ½ tsp hot chilli flakes, or a few dashes Tabasco)

Rind and juice of 1 fresh lemon

Plenty of freshly ground black pepper

½ cup/generous handful toasted pine nuts, to garnish

Fresh salad leaves, to serve

Heat the olive oil over a medium heat in a medium-sized saucepan. Add the red onion and sweat for a few minutes, then stir in the garlic and cumin and cook for another minute or so. Add the stock and bring to the boil. Take the pan off the heat and add the bulgur wheat. Cover the pan and leave it for 10 minutes until the bulgur has absorbed all the liquid. Tip the bulgur into a bowl and stir in the tomatoes, butter beans, herbs, chilli, lemon juice, lemon rind and pepper. Allow to cool, then refrigerate for an hour or so before serving to allow the flavours to develop. 'Fluff' with a fork, sprinkle with toasted pine nuts and serve with crisp salad leaves and houmous. Great for lunch boxes.

Nutty Chickpea and Sesame 'Burgers'

Preparation time: 20 minutes, Chilling time: 40–60 minutes, Cooking time: 5 minutes, Makes 10–12 small 'burgers'

820g/4 cups chickpeas, drained

2 tbsp sesame oil

2 tbsp tahini paste

Large handful mint, finely chopped (approximately 2 tbsp)

1 tbsp extra virgin olive oil or avocado oil

Zest of ½ a lemon

Juice of 2 lemons

100g/1 cup walnut pieces

50g/¾ cup ground almonds

100g/1 cup sunflower seeds

100% wholemeal flour for dusting (or spelt, buckwheat or rye
    flour – whatever you have)

2 medium free-range eggs, beaten

Put the chickpeas, sesame oil, tahini paste, mint, olive oil, lemon zest and juice into a food processor and blend to a smooth paste. Chop the nuts and sunflower seeds until quite fine. Dust your hands with flour and form small burgers with the chickpea mixture. Roll them in a little flour, dip in the egg and then coat in nuts. Refrigerate for an hour before cooking. Then cook for 5 minutes under the grill or in a frying pan with the smallest amount of oil. They also barbecue brilliantly! Serve with a crisp salad or low-GL veggies. Great lunch-box stand-bys.

Lentil and Tomato Salad

Preparation time: 10 minutes, Cooking time: 30 minutes, Serves 4

225g/1 cup green (or red) lentils

1 medium onion, chopped

1 clove garlic, chopped roughly (optional)

1 small red chilli pepper, deseeded and diced

900ml/4 cups water

1 bay leaf

4 tbsp extra virgin olive oil

2 tbsp balsamic vinegar

Juice of ½ a lemon

225g/1 cup chopped tomatoes

1 large red pepper, singed, peeled and roughly chopped (or
    use the ones that come in oil in tins or jars)

4 spring onions, chopped

15/½ cup black olives, stoned and chopped roughly

2 tbsp fresh parsley, chopped

Put the lentils and onion into a pan with the garlic (if desired) and the chilli pepper. Pour in the water and add the bay leaf. Bring to the boil, cover and simmer for about 30 minutes (or as per packet instructions) until tender. Drain, rinse and remove the bay leaf. Put the mixture into a large salad bowl and allow to cool. Pour over the olive oil, balsamic vinegar and lemon juice, then add all the remaining ingredients, toss well and serve.

Zesty Vegetable Kebabs with Wild Rice and Chickpeas

Preparation time: 15 minutes, Marinating time: 10 minutes minimum, Cooking time: 5 minutes, Serves 2

Marinade
1 small red chilli, deseeded and chopped finely
Zest and juice of 2 limes (or lemons)
Zest and juice of 1 orange
2 tbsp extra virgin olive oil
1 tsp fructose or honey
½ tsp paprika
½ tsp ground coriander

Kebabs
Use a selection of your favourite veggies, preferably baby
    ones, such as: courgettes (zucchini), cherry tomatoes,
    baby onions or shallots (scallions) or normal onions cut
    into quarters

plus:
250g pack halloumi cheese, cut into chunks about 1 inch
    (3cm) square
Red peppers
Button mushrooms

Wild rice and chickpeas

3 tbsp extra virgin olive oil

1 clove garlic, grated or crushed

200g/1 cup chickpeas, drained and rinsed

150g/¾ cup (1 handful) wild rice

2 large handfuls fresh baby spinach (or herbs), chopped roughly

To serve

Lemon wedges

Freshly ground black pepper

Blend the marinade ingredients. Toss all the veg and halloumi in the marinade, making sure it's all covered. Marinade for up to 2 hours (at least 10 minutes).

Meanwhile, take a handful of wild rice, put into a pot of boiling water and simmer for approximately 40 minutes (or as per packet instructions). When done, drain and rinse with cold water.

Put 1 tbsp olive oil in a pan over a medium heat. Add the garlic, allow to cook gently for a minute at most, then add the cooked wild rice and chickpeas. Toss these in the garlicky oil, allow to warm through, then turn off the heat and leave to sit.

Thread the marinated veggies and halloumi onto skewers (soak wooden skewers in water while the veg is marinating), then grill, griddle or barbecue for about 5 minutes. Stir the fresh spinach through the wild rice and chickpea mix, and divide this between the plates. Put the kebabs on top. Serve with lemon wedges and plenty of freshly ground black pepper. When cold, this makes a great lunch-box option.

Curried Butternut Squash Soup

Preparation time: 15 minutes, Cooking time: 20–30 minutes, Serves 6, Freezes well

1 large butternut squash (or pumpkin or other squash)

1 cooking apple

35g/2tbsp butter or olive oil-based spread

1 onion, diced

2 garlic cloves, grated or crushed

1–2 tsp curry powder (to your taste)

1 litre/4 cups vegetable stock

Freshly ground black pepper

To serve

5 tbsp natural yoghurt/crème fraîche

1 tsp horseradish

1 tsp curry powder

2 sprigs mint, chopped roughly, to garnish

Peel and deseed the squash/pumpkin. Peel, core and chop the apple. Heat the butter in a large pan, add the onion and sweat for 4–5 minutes. Add the garlic and curry powder and stir for 2 minutes. Add the squash, apple and stock, bring to the boil, then simmer for 20–30 minutes until soft. Purée in a blender, return to the pan and season to taste. Don't boil again.

Serve with horseradish cream: mix the yoghurt or crème fraîche with the horseradish and curry powder. Stir a tablespoonful into each bowl of soup and sprinkle with mint. This freezes really well.

Asparagus, Lemon and Mint 'Barleyotto'

Preparation time: 10 minutes, Cooking time: 40 minutes, Serves 4

Pearl barley is an excellent substitute for rice in risotto-style dishes.

25g/2 tbsp butter or olive oil-based spread

1 medium onion or 3 shallots, diced

2–3 cloves garlic, grated or crushed

100ml/½ cup dry white wine

200g/1 cup pearl barley

700ml/3 cups chicken stock

500g fresh asparagus (discard any woody bits, chop into
    smallish chunks and boil lightly until cooked but still *al
    dente*)

Zest of 1 lemon

Juice of ½ a lemon

Good handful chopped fresh mint (about 4 tbsp once
    chopped)

To serve

40g/¼ cup pine nuts or chopped walnuts

Lemon wedges

Freshly ground black pepper

Melt the butter or olive oil-based spread in a large pan over a medium heat. Add the onion, stir-frying gently for about a minute, then add the garlic and cook for a further minute, being careful not to let the garlic burn. Pour in the wine to deglaze the pan, turn up the heat and bring to the boil. Boil for 4–5 minutes, stirring until it reaches the consistency of syrup. Turn down the heat and add the barley, then put in about a third of the chicken stock, stirring all the time. Once it is starting to be absorbed, pour in the rest of the stock, and cook until all is absorbed, about 35–40 minutes. Keep an eye on it and stir regularly.

If you are using pine nuts, put them in a small dry pan and toast until golden. They burn easily so be careful. Stir in the asparagus, grate over the lemon zest, sprinkle with mint, squeeze over the lemon juice and stir.

Grind over fresh black pepper, sprinkle with pine nuts and serve with lemon wedges.

Bean Sprout Salad

Mention sprouting seeds and many folk think we're bark-ing mad. These little darlings pack a punch, however, and add a really zingy freshness to any salad. You can either sprout your fave seeds in a jam jar (remember how much fun growing mustard and cress was at school?!) or you can get serious with a sprouter (available from most health-food shops) and a good mix of edible seeds. Don't panic – you can also buy them ready sprouted in most supermar-kets and health-food shops!

Sprouted seeds keep in the fridge in a bag for a couple of days, but are best eaten fresh. Harvest when just sprouted (tastiest time), squeeze over half a lemon and a tablespoon of olive oil. They're delicious as a snack with some houmous. They also taste great under a thin layer of melted cheese on top of low-GL bread … yum!

Avocado, Tomato, Mozzarella and Spinach Salad

Preparation time: 10 minutes, Serves 6 as starter/side dish, 2–3 as a main course

½ bag fresh baby spinach leaves, rinsed and chopped roughly
2 avocados, peeled and sliced
6 big, flavoursome tomatoes, sliced thinly
1 buffalo mozzarella, sliced
2 large handfuls fresh basil, torn roughly
1 tbsp balsamic vinegar
Juice of ½ a lemon
4 tbsp extra virgin olive oil
Freshly ground black pepper

Put the spinach on a big platter (or individual plates or a lunchbox). Arrange the avocados, tomatoes and mozzarella on top. Sprinkle with basil and pour over the balsamic vinegar, lemon juice and olive oil. Grind plenty of fresh black pepper over the salad and serve.

'Lemon Heaven'

Preparation time: 5 minutes, Refrigeration time: 30 minutes, Serves 2

1 tbsp fructose
125ml/1 cup natural yoghurt
Juice of ½ lemon
Zest of 1 lemon or mint sprigs, to garnish

Put the fructose in a coffee grinder and whizz until it has an 'icing sugar' consistency. Stir it into the yoghurt and mix in the lemon juice. Transfer to small cups, refrigerate, add a decorative curl of lemon zest or sprig of mint to each before serving. These make brilliant snack pots.

Avocado and Tomato Pot

Preparation time: 10 minutes, Serves 1

1 avocado, diced
2 tomatoes, diced
Generous handful fresh basil, chopped roughly
1 tbsp extra virgin olive oil
1 tbsp balsamic vinegar
Squeeze of lemon
Generous grating of Parmesan cheese

Mix all the ingredients together, put in a small pot or bowl and bingo – really tasty lunch! Lovely with a couple of oatcakes.

Toasted Courgette, Garlic and Basil Pasta

Preparation time: 5 minutes for the sauce, Cooking time: 20 minutes plus pasta cooking time, Serves 4

500g courgettes (zucchini), sliced thickly

4 tbsp extra virgin olive oil

320–350g wholewheat pasta (you are aiming for 100g cooked-weight pasta per person – see the food lists in Chapter 10)

4 garlic cloves, chopped, grated or crushed

4 tsp sun-dried tomato paste

2 tsp balsamic vinegar (Worcester sauce works well too!)

Good handful chopped fresh basil (about 4 tbsp once chopped)

1 cup/generous handful black olives, pitted and chopped roughly

Freshly ground black pepper

To serve

Grated Parmesan or Cheddar

Basil sprigs

Heat the oven to 230°C/450°F/Gas Mark 8. Toss the courgettes in 2 tbsp olive oil, put onto a baking tray and bake for 20 minutes until golden and tender (take care not to burn). Cook the pasta until *al dente* with the garlic added to the water. Drain the pasta, return it to the pan and toss in the remaining olive oil, sun-dried tomato paste and balsamic vinegar. Add the courgettes to the mixture along with any pan juices, the basil, olives and freshly ground black pepper. Grate over some Parmesan or Cheddar and serve garnished with basil sprigs.

Mushrooms on Low-GL Toast

Preparation time: 5 minutes, Cooking time: 10 minutes, Serves 2

25g butter/2 tbsp olive oil-based spread

2 cups mushrooms, sliced

1–2 cloves garlic, grated or crushed

4 tbsp crème fraîche/sour cream

1 tsp grainy mustard

2 pieces low-GL toast

Fresh chives, to garnish

Freshly ground black pepper

Heat the butter or spread in a pan over a medium heat. Add the mushrooms and stir. Cook for about 5 minutes, stir the garlic into the mushrooms and cook for another couple of minutes. Remove from the heat and stir in the crème fraîche and mustard. Pile onto low-GL toast, snip chives over the top, and grind over plenty of fresh black pepper.

Vegetables 'Greek Style'

**Preparation time: 15 minutes, Cooking time: 35–40 minutes,
Serves 4 as a side dish**

4 tomatoes, sliced thinly
1 aubergine (eggplant), cut into cubes
½ bag (2 large handfuls) baby spinach, washed and chopped
    (or use the freezer blocks of spinach – allow to thaw
    enough to incorporate into the mix)
3 sticks celery, sliced
1 medium onion, sliced
1 red pepper, deseeded and sliced
Juice and zest of 1 lemon
4 tbsp extra virgin olive oil
Big handful of your favourite fresh herb – coriander (cilantro),
    basil, mint
2 tbsp fresh rosemary, off the stalk and roughly chopped
Plenty of freshly ground black pepper
120g/¾ cup feta cheese
Generous handful black olives, pitted and roughly chopped

Preheat the oven to 200°C/400°F/Gas Mark 6. Arrange
half the sliced tomatoes in the bottom of a non-stick
baking dish. Mix the remaining tomatoes with the rest of
the vegetables, lemon and oil, fresh herbs, rosemary and a
generous grinding of black pepper in a bowl and spoon
over the tomato slices. Cover and bake for 30 minutes,
until the veg is *al dente*. Uncover, sprinkle with feta cheese
and olives and bake for a further 5–10 minutes.

Butterbean and Avocado Salad with Heavenly Grilled Pepper Dressing*

Preparation time: 20 minutes, Serves 2

For the salad

1 bag mixed salad leaves

1 avocado, cut into chunks

1 can (usually 410g)/2 cups butter beans, drained and rinsed

Fresh Parmesan shavings

For the dressing

1 red pepper (or red peppers in jars of olive oil for ease)

1 orange or yellow pepper (as above)

1–2 cloves garlic, grated or crushed

4 tbsp/50ml white wine vinegar

250ml/1 cup extra virgin olive oil

Freshly ground black pepper

* You can use a shop-bought dressing instead.

To prepare the dressing, singe the red and yellow or orange peppers under the grill. Put them in a bag, leave for a few minutes then peel off the skin and discard the stalk and seeds. Alternatively, drain the oil from the peppers in the jar (keep the oil; use it instead of the olive oil). Put the peppers in a blender with the garlic and vinegar and blend until smooth. Transfer to a bowl and gently stir in the olive oil. The dressing is good blended or 'separated' – in fact, it looks better when it separates. This is also a great dressing for bulgur wheat or other beans as a side dish.

Put the salad leaves, avocado and butter beans in a large salad bowl, drench with the dressing and toss until covered. Grind over some black pepper and shave/grate over some Parmesan.

This makes a delicious side salad too.

Tomato and Cauli 'Crumble'

Preparation time: 10 minutes, Cooking time: 30 minutes, Serves 4

1 medium cauliflower head, cut/broken into florets

2 cloves garlic, chopped roughly

6 tomatoes, sliced

1 tsp fresh thyme leaves, chopped (oregano also works well)

25g olive oil-based spread or butter

For the crumble

50g/½ cup spelt/rye/100% wholemeal flour

50g/¾ cup ground almonds

225g/1 cup old-fashioned porridge oats

50g/½ cup mature Cheddar, grated

3 cloves garlic, grated or crushed

Freshly ground black pepper

4 tbsp butter or olive oil-based spread

Preheat the oven to 200°C/400°F/Gas Mark 6. Boil or steam the cauliflower with the garlic in the water until almost cooked but still crisp. Drain well (cauliflower holds water like a sponge!). Pack tightly into a lightly oiled baking dish, cover with the tomato slices, sprinkle with thyme, dot with spread/butter and liberally grind over fresh black pepper.

In a large bowl mix together the flour, almonds, oats, cheese, crushed garlic and seasoning. Gently melt the butter/spread in a small pan, and then stir into the crumble mixture. It should be crumbly! Sprinkle it evenly over the top of the cauli/tomato mixture. Bake for about 30 minutes until crisp and golden brown. Serve immediately with lightly steamed greens tossed in chilli.

❝ I really piled the weight on when pregnant due to an unhealthy diet and a craving for milk shakes! After the birth of my daughter, it took me a long time to lose the initial 3st by the GI diet alone. After being stuck at a weight-loss plateau for weeks, I heard about the GL diet. It made so much more sense so I switched and was surprised how the last half a stone just 'fell off'! Within a month I was back in my size 10 jeans! It was so easy and the recipes were so delicious – no 'diet' food in sight! The lack of hunger pangs between meals was really noticeable, and I had no more sugar cravings. I was also very pleased to see that Diet Freedom had a website with a wonderful forum. This is a source of so much support and encouragement, not only from fellow readers, but also from the team themselves. They make you very welcome and there's always someone there to chat to, share recipes with and buddy up with if you want to. ❞

Caroline P from Rainham, Kent

Chapter 8

THE 7-DAY FOODIE FRIENDLY PLAN

This plan assumes you have a real inclination to cook and the time to prepare a few things in advance for your new low-GL foodie-friendly lifestyle.

This is good food, not diet food! The recipes serve more than one as we're assuming you'll want to share share share with loved ones. Many of the breakfast and lunch options make enough for a couple of meals.

I've got a real thing for fresh herbs and fresh ingredients in general. My spice rack is heaving with dried and powdered herbs and ready-made spice blends – I'm not a purist, rather a taste-ist.

Where any recipe calls for fresh herbs, garlic or ginger, you can use the dried versions. It alters the taste a little, but will still be delicious.

There's garlic in quite a lot of the recipes – because it's just heavenly and so good for you – but please feel free to omit it if you're eating at the office and would like to remain on good terms with your colleagues! Chilli, again, is optional. Often it is added for warmth rather than taste, so do add or subtract it to suit your palate or location.

Herbs and spices can lift a dish to dizzying heights and have some great health properties too. Please do experiment with them. There is no added salt in any of these recipes, and again this is where the herbs and spices come in to their own.

When we suggest serving a recipe with low-GL veggies, please choose your favourites. We have also included some great veggie side-dish recipes.

When salad is recommended with a meal, please don't envisage the nasty soggy lettuce of the rabbit-diet days. Go mad with your leaves. Include lots of fresh herbs and leaves such as rocket, spinach and watercress. Lettuce need not be your only leaf.

Tina and Nigel look at me like I'm mad because I grow some of my own salad vegetables. My 'easy gardening' includes rocket, basil, all flavours of mint, nasturtiums (gorgeously peppery edible flowers), chives, sage, thyme, and the 'everlasting lettuce' (where you pick the leaves you want and it keeps on growing!). I'm no great gardener – these are all in pots – but these few things keep us in fresh leaves that are quite expensive to buy in the shops at the cost of only a packet or two of seeds and the occasional bit of watering.

Lemon and lime juice are other secret taste-boosters that add an intense zing to most dishes, not just fish. They have the added bonus of allegedly lowering the glycaemic impact of the meal, so get squeezing!

I'm a fairly lazy cook, truth be told. However, cooking is my 'meditation' and it does help me wind down at the end of a hectic day. Of course there are days when the time/energy factor is not there and I am *so* pleased to have Tina's swift and delicious recipes to hand too – so do mix and match plans and recipes depending on your energy and enthusiasm level!

For a shopping list for this plan, please see Chapter 11 (pages 228–34).

Lastly, don't be put off by a bit more time and preparation. You deserve the time and effort spent on you, so go on … treat yourself!

Where oatcakes/crispbreads or slices of bread are mentioned in the plan, men should have up to 4 oatcakes crispbreads or 2 slices of bread; women should have up to 2 oatcakes/crispbreads or 1 slice of bread.

Eating regularly – every four hours – is important to help balance your blood sugar levels so try not to skip meals and snacks.

	Day 1	Day 2	Day 3	Day 4	Day 5	Day 6	Day 7
Breakfast	*Diet Freedom Muesli	*Summer Berries with Greek Yoghurt	Half a papaya (pawpaw) with freshly squeezed lime juice	*Nutty Seedy Bread with sugar-free peanut butter	*Diet Freedom Muesli	*Greek-style Yoghurt with Nuts, Seeds, Mint and Fresh Ginger	*Scrambled Eggs with Smoked Salmon
Snack	*Herby Guacamole and crudités	*Diet Freedom Toasted Seed Mix with dried apricots	*Melon and Mint Fruit Salad	1 sliced apple with piece of cheese	*Diet Freedom Toasted Seed Mix	*Herby Cream Cheese with crudités	Oatcakes with *Houmous
Lunch	*Marinated Feta Cheese with *Nutty Seedy Bread and olives	*Chickpea and Pepper Salad	*Smoked Mackerel Pâté with oatcakes and salad	*Chunky Bean and Bacon Soup	*Roasted Vegetable, Bean and Bulgur Wheat Salad	*Pea and Mint Soup with *Nutty Seed Bread	*Giant Prawns with Mucho-spicy Dip and Salad

	Day 1	Day 2	Day 3	Day 4	Day 5	Day 6	Day 7
Snack	1 sliced nectarine	Few squares (about 25g) chocolate (at least 70% cocoa)	*Diet Freedom Toasted Seed Mix	Oatcakes with *Tzatziki	*Goat's Cheese with Pear	*Diet Freedom Toasted Seed Mix	Handful of grapes
Dinner	*Tuna Steak with Tomato and Basil Sauce plus low-GL veggies	*Spicy Meatballs with Tomato Sauce plus low-GL veggies	*Chilli, Lime and Ginger Chicken plus low-GL veggies	*Grilled Hoki with Rocket and Sun-dried Tomato Salad	*Red pepper, Chorizo and Basil 'Barleyotto'	*Beef and Vegetable Casserole plus low-GL veggies	*Pea and Mint Soup with *Nutty Seedy Bread

* Recipes for these dishes are given in the following pages.

Diet Freedom Muesli

Preparation time: 10 minutes

We've used cups not weights in this recipe as you can use any measure (cup, mug, etc.) and keep the ratio the same, or substitute different ingredients that have different weights. To make up a bigger batch, just scale up all the ingredients equally.

2 cups old-fashioned porridge oats (don't use the
    microwaveable quick-cook ones)
¼ cup sunflower seeds
¼ cup linseeds
¼ cup pumpkin seeds
½ cup nut pieces – hazelnuts, almonds, brazil nuts,
    macadamias or walnuts (or a mixture)
½ cup unsweetened coconut flakes/desiccated coconut
2 tsp cinnamon powder
1 cup sugar-free bran sticks

If you like your muesli 'toasted' follow the instructions below – if not, you can just mix all the ingredients together.

Mix all the above ingredients (except the bran sticks) in a baking tray. Bake in a hot oven (200°C/400°F/Gas Mark 6) for approximately 15 minutes, until lightly 'toasted' and the oats have turned golden at the edges. Carefully remove from the oven and allow to cool. Once cooled, place the toasted ingredients with the bran sticks in a storage jar and shake until mixed well. Adding the dried or fresh fruit below will 'sweeten' the muesli without the need for added sugar, although you could sprinkle with a teaspoon of fructose if you prefer it sweeter. Serve with skimmed milk or unsweetened soya milk.

Optional Extras
- $1/2$ cup oat bran
- $1/2$ cup chopped dried apricots, dried apples or dried strawberries
- Chop in some fresh low-GL fruit just before serving

Herby Guacamole

Preparation time: 10 minutes, Serves 2

Big handful fresh coriander (cilantro) or basil
1 clove garlic (optional)
1 tsp freshly ground black pepper
Dash of Tabasco or a pinch of chilli powder (to your taste)
15ml/1 tbsp lemon juice
2 tbsp extra virgin olive oil
2 avocados

Put the coriander, garlic, pepper and Tabasco or chilli into a blender and whizz. (If you don't have a blender, mash with a fork.) Add half the lemon juice and whizz again, then slowly add the olive oil as the blender combines the ingredients. Peel and stone the avocados, add the flesh to the blender and pulse until blended in but still chunky, then stir in the rest of the lemon juice. Garnish with a dash of paprika and serve with crudités.

Marinated Feta Cheese

Preparation time: 15 minutes, Makes 6–8 servings

350g/2 cups feta cheese
1 garlic clove, sliced
1 tsp mixed peppercorns (or black)
2 bay leaves
1 tsp coriander seeds, crushed
2 tsp capers (in brine, drained)
4 sprigs fresh thyme or 1 tsp dried
Extra virgin olive oil to cover

Cut the feta into chunks and layer in a clean jar with the herbs and spices. Cover with olive oil, close and leave to mature in the fridge for up to a week. This is a fabulous topper for salads – almost a chunky dressing. It's also good with oatcakes, olives and a sliced apple for lunch or on low-GL toast. Serve with lemon wedges, squeezed over. Don't keep for more than a week.

Variations
Add some olives and a pinch of chilli to the mix

Nutty Seedy Bread

Preparation time: 10 minutes, Cooking time: depends on your bread machine, 10–12 slices per loaf

This is quite a dense, nutty loaf, and is best for 'open' sandwiches.

¾ tsp yeast (dried/fast active – specifically for bread machines)

200g 100% wholemeal stone-ground flour/bread flour

150g spelt flour (or rye flour)

50g old-fashioned porridge oats (or rye flakes or buckwheat flakes)

1 tbsp fructose/honey/sugar *(sugar feeds the yeast)*

1 tbsp olive oil

1 tsp salt *(an important part of the yeast/sugar balance)*

¾ tsp vitamin C powder

7 tbsp linseeds or flax seeds (or 7 tbsp Diet Freedom's Toasted Seed Mix, page 121)

3 tbsp crushed nuts – walnuts, almonds, brazils, hazelnuts, etc.

300ml water + 1 tbsp milk (if you are doing your bread on an overnight setting then use milk powder as the milk may sour, and add another tablespoon of water)

Make the bread according to your bread machine's instructions – generally on the 'wholemeal' setting.

Note: We haven't used cup equivalents in the measurements because it is important to be exact in bread making.

Tuna Steaks with Tomato and Basil Sauce

Preparation time: 10 minutes, Cooking time: 15 minutes, Serves 4

1 tbsp extra virgin olive oil

1 onion, diced

3 cloves garlic, crushed or grated

1 tin (usually about 400g/2 cups) chopped tomatoes in their
   juice

1 small pinch chilli powder or 2 dashes Tabasco sauce (for
   warmth, not taste)

Freshly ground black pepper

4 tuna steaks (works with other fish too, such as salmon and
   hoki)

Generous handful fresh basil, roughly chopped

½ cup/generous handful pine nuts

3 spring onions, chopped

Preheat the oven to 180°C/350°F/Gas Mark 4. Heat the olive oil over a medium heat in a medium-sized saucepan. Add the onion and fry gently for a minute or so. Add the garlic, fry for about 30 seconds then add the tomatoes. Sprinkle in the chilli powder or Tabasco and add a generous grinding of black pepper. Simmer for 10–15 minutes. Then liquidize (unless you like a chunky sauce), return to the pan and bubble quickly for another 5 minutes or so until reduced. Remove from the heat and allow to cool slightly.

Put each tuna steak in an oiled piece of aluminium foil big enough to fold up completely around the fish and sauce. Stir most of the basil into the sauce. Divide the sauce between the steaks then wrap up the foil parcels (roughly pinch the edges together to make as airtight as possible). Bake on a baking tray for 10–15 minutes.

Toss the pine nuts in a small dry frying pan until golden, taking care not to burn them, then take off the heat. Carefully transfer each tuna steak in its foil parcel onto a plate and open (mind the steam), sprinkle with spring onions, pine nuts and the remaining chopped basil. Serve immediately with low-GL vegetables.

If you have a favourite tomato-based sauce that comes in a jar and is low-GL, make it even simpler by using that!

Summer Berries with Greek Yoghurt

Preparation time: 4 minutes, Serves 1

This works with any low-GL fruit, and is great with a sprinkling of Toasted Seed Mix too (see page 121). If you find
Greek yoghurt too rich, use half the quantity and half
natural bio yoghurt to make it creamy but a little less
intense.

2 cups/generous handfuls summer berries (Choose your
    favourites. If out of season, buy frozen berries and take
    what you need out of the freezer the night before. By
    morning they will be thawed, squidgy and delicious!)
250 ml/1 cup Greek yoghurt

Stir the berries and yoghurt together and drizzle with $\frac{1}{2}$
tsp honey or sprinkle with fructose if needed. Lovely
breakfast!

Diet Freedom's Toasted Seed Mix

Preparation time: 5 minutes, Cooking time: 10–15 minutes, Makes 8–10 servings

Use a cup, mug or whatever to measure the ingredients, and substitute or add other seeds and nuts to the mix as you wish. Bear in mind that nuts are calorie dense, so check the food lists in Chapter 10 and generally stick to 1 cup/measure per mix.

1 cup linseeds/flax seeds

1 cup sunflower seeds

1 cup pumpkin seeds

½ cup sesame seeds

½ cup pine nuts

1 cup unsweetened desiccated coconut

1 tsp cinnamon powder (optional)

Put all the ingredients in a big dry frying pan on a high heat until you hear the seeds start to 'pop', then turn the heat down to medium. Keep the seeds moving as they will burn easily. Once they are golden in colour turn off the heat.

These are great on top of yoghurt. You could also try a couple of handfuls with a few dried apricots as a snack, or use as a crunchy topping for salads.

Spicy Meatballs with Tomato Sauce

Preparation time: 20 minutes, Cooking time: 30 minutes, Serves 4

3 tbsp pine nuts

6 tbsp extra virgin olive oil

1 large onion, finely diced

3 cloves garlic, grated or crushed

2 tsp ground cumin

1 tsp ground cardamom

1½ tsp chilli flakes or chilli powder

1 tsp ground allspice

Large bunch coriander (cilantro), washed, drained and
    chopped very finely

Freshly ground black pepper

600g/4½ cups minced beef (also works with lamb or poultry)

Tomato sauce

1 large onion, diced

4 cloves garlic, grated or crushed

1 can (approximately 400g/2 cups) chopped tomatoes or
    passata (sieved tomatoes)

1 tbsp Worcester sauce

Plenty of freshly ground black pepper

Lightly toast the pine nuts in a dry pan then transfer to a large mixing bowl. Heat a tbsp or so of the olive oil in the pan and sweat the finely diced onions. Add the garlic, cumin, cardamom, chilli and allspice, cook for another minute or so and then add to the mixing bowl. Add the coriander, the seasoning and the meat. Mulch it all together with clean fingers. Roll into meatballs – you should get about 16 from this mix – or if you prefer, squash into small 'patties' or burgers. Put on a plate as you go along, cover with cling film and chill for 10 minutes (up to 24 hours) until firm. (These freeze really well).

To make the sauce, fry the onion in a large pan, add the garlic about 2 minutes later, then tomatoes, Worcester sauce and seasoning. Cook for 10 minutes. If you like a smooth sauce, use passata instead of chopped tomatoes, or at this point put the sauce through a blender and return to the pan. Taste – it should be fairly bland as the meatballs are pretty spicy! Allow to simmer and reduce as you cook the meatballs.

Fry or grill the meatballs until cooked through (around 7–10 minutes). Serve with the tomato sauce, a wedge of lemon and a salad or low-GL veggies.

Chickpea and Pepper Salad

Preparation time: 5–10 minutes, Cooking time: 10–15 minutes, Serves 2

2 tbsp extra virgin olive oil

Pinch of chilli powder, dash of Tabasco or ½ tsp chilli flakes –
    depending on your preference

2 cardamom pods, pod removed and seeds crushed

1 red onion, sliced thinly

2 cloves garlic, crushed or grated (optional)

1 red pepper, skinned, deseeded and sliced into chunky strips
    (or a couple of prepared peppers from a jar in olive oil)

1 can chickpeas (approx 410g/2 cups), drained and rinsed

Plenty of freshly ground black pepper to taste

Heat the olive oil in a pan over a medium heat, add the spices and onion and sweat for a couple of minutes. Stir in the garlic, red pepper and chickpeas. Allow to cook for about 10 minutes, then taste and season. Serve as a side salad or a vegetable side dish. Alternatively, allow to cool and eat as a lunchtime salad, stirring in some rocket and maybe grating over a little Parmesan.

Melon and Mint Fruit Salad

Preparation time: 5 minutes, Serves 2

½ medium-sized melon (any type, including watermelon – if
    out of season you can buy frozen melon balls in the freezer
    section and transfer to the fridge the day before you need
    them)
Generous handful of mint

Chop the melon into chunks and toss in a bowl with the
mint – a really zingy refreshing snack or breakfast.

Smoked Mackerel Pâté

Preparation time: 10 minutes, Serves 2

1 packet smoked mackerel
250ml/1 cup Greek-style yoghurt (or cream cheese/half-fat
    cream cheese)
Plenty of freshly ground black pepper
Rind of 1 fresh lemon
1 tbsp fresh lemon juice

Take the skin off the mackerel fillets and break the flesh
into a bowl. Remove any stray bones. Add in the rest of the
ingredients and mash together. Serve as a dip with crudités
or for lunch with oatcakes and salad or on toasted low-GL
bread.

Chilli, Lime and Ginger Chicken

**Preparation time: 10 minutes, Chilling time: 2–24 hours,
Cooking time: 15–20 minutes, Serves 4**

300ml/1½ cups coconut milk (from a tin, a block or the
    powdered version – follow packet instructions)
1 hot red chilli, deseeded and diced finely (or 1 tsp chilli
    flakes/powder)
1-inch/3cm piece fresh ginger, grated finely
Zest and juice of 1 lime
1 tsp coriander seeds, crushed
2 tbsp fresh coriander (cilantro), chopped finely
4 large skinless chicken breasts

Put all the ingredients except the chicken in a large, sturdy
freezer bag. Then add the chicken breasts and squish and
squelch until you are sure all the chicken has a good
covering. Seal the bag, place in a bowl and refrigerate for
at least 2 hours (preferably for 24 hours).

When you're ready to cook, heat the grill to maximum
and grill the chicken for 6–10 minutes each side. The
cooking time depends on the size of the chicken breasts
and how hot your grill is – the chicken is cooked if the
juices run clear when you poke the thickest bit with a knife
or skewer. Serve with low-GL veggies or a big crispy salad.

Chunky Bean and Bacon Soup

Preparation time: 15 minutes, Cooking time: 20 minutes, Serves 4

If you're taking this for lunch in a Thermos, leave out the croutons – too soggy! Take a slice of the low-GL bread, spread it with goat's cheese and get dippy with it instead.

2 tbsp extra virgin olive oil

50g/½ cup smoky bacon or chorizo/salami, diced finely

3 cloves garlic, diced

½ tsp chilli flakes or pinch of chilli powder (for warmth, not taste)

820g/4 cups in total of cannellini, haricot, butter beans or chickpeas – or a mix of each (these usually come in 410g tins), drained and rinsed

900ml/4 cups water or stock

Freshly ground black pepper

3 generous handfuls shredded cabbage – the dark-green variety is most striking!

2 tbsp finely chopped parsley, coriander (cilantro) or basil

2 slices low-GL bread (such as Nutty Seedy Bread, page 116)

40g/1 cup mature Cheddar, grated

More fresh herbs, to garnish

Put a large, heavy-bottomed pan over a medium heat and add 1 tbsp olive oil. Add the bacon and cook for about 3 minutes, then add the garlic and chilli and stir in for about a minute. Add the beans and water/stock and bring to the boil. At this point liquidize half the soup mixture and return it to the pan. Season generously and simmer for another 5 minutes or so.

Meanwhile, toast the low-GL bread, sprinkle with the mature Cheddar (or spread with soft goat's cheese) and put under a hot grill for a few minutes. Remove, and cut into quarters. Add the cabbage to the soup and simmer for another couple of minutes. Stir in the fresh chopped herbs, divide the soup between 4 bowls, add the cheesy croutons and sprinkle with fresh herbs. Serve hot.

Tzatziki/Raita

Preparation time: 10 minutes, Serves 2–4

250ml/1 cup natural Greek yoghurt (for tzatziki), bio yoghurt
(for raita)
3 tbsp finely chopped mint
2 tbsp lemon juice
½ cucumber, peeled, deseeded and finely chopped
Freshly ground black pepper to taste

Mix all the ingredients together and chill. Serve as a dip with crudités or with oatcakes (tzatziki), as an accompaniment to hot and spicy dishes (raita) or as a salad dressing.

Grilled Hoki with Rocket and Sun-dried Tomato Salad

Preparation time: 10 minutes, Cooking time: 10 minutes, Serves 2

2 hoki fillets (works with all fish)

2 tbsp sun-dried tomato oil (or olive oil)

Freshly ground black pepper

1 bag rocket or mixed salad leaves

5–8 sun-dried tomatoes (preferably preserved in olive oil),
    drained and chopped roughly

8–10 olives, pitted and chopped roughly

2 tbsp balsamic vinegar

Juice of ½ a lemon

Brush the hoki fillets with some of the sun-dried tomato oil (or olive oil), and generously grind over some fresh black pepper. Put under a medium-to-hot grill and cook for around 7–10 minutes, depending on the heat of your grill, turning once.

Wash the salad, drain and arrange the leaves on a plate. Sprinkle with sun-dried tomatoes and olives, then dress with balsamic vinegar and sun-dried tomato or olive oil. When cooked, put the hoki on top of the salad, squeeze over the lemon juice and serve.

Roasted Vegetable, Bean and Bulgur Wheat Salad

Preparation time: 5 minutes, Cooking time: 30 minutes, Serves 4 as a side salad

1 bulb fennel, washed and sliced chunkily

2 red/orange peppers, deseeded and sliced chunkily

1 red onion, sliced chunkily

2 sprigs rosemary, off stalks

1 tsp paprika

2 cloves garlic, grated or crushed

3 tbsp extra virgin olive oil

2 tbsp balsamic vinegar

200g/1 cup bulgur wheat

250g/1½ cups butter beans, drained and rinsed

4 artichoke hearts, cut into quarters (optional)

Freshly ground black pepper

1 bag rocket/watercress, chopped roughly

Preheat the oven to 200°C/400°F/Gas Mark 6. Put all the veg in a baking dish, snip the rosemary leaves over and sprinkle with paprika and garlic. Pour over the olive oil and balsamic vinegar and toss the veg so all are covered. Put into the oven and cook until tender, with some crispy edges – about 20–25 minutes.

Cook the bulgur wheat as per the packet instructions, then drain. Put the bulgur wheat and butter beans in a large salad bowl. Pour in the hot veg and any juice, and add the artichoke hearts if using. Season with plenty of black pepper. Toss with the rocket or watercress, so all are combined. Serve immediately as a side salad to accompany any grilled meat or as a main salad with some raita/tzatziki (see page 130). For a packed lunch, leave out the rocket and watercress (it will go soggy). Take it in a separate bag and combine just before eating.

Red Pepper, Chorizo and Basil 'Barleyotto'

Preparation time: 10 minutes, Cooking time: 45 minutes, Serves 4–6

25g/2 tbsp butter or olive oil-based spread

1 tsp extra virgin olive oil

1 medium onion or 3 shallots, diced

2–3 cloves garlic, grated or crushed

100ml/½ cup dry white wine

700ml/3 cups chicken stock

200g/1 cup pearl barley

100g/1 cup roughly chopped chorizo (or lean bacon as a
    lower-fat alternative)

2 red peppers, skinned and chopped (or use peppers in jars
    of olive oil)

Freshly ground black pepper

1 big handful fresh basil, chopped roughly

Melt the butter or spread and the olive oil in a large pan on a medium heat. Add the onion and fry for about a minute, stirring gently, then add the garlic and cook for just another minute, taking care not to let the garlic burn. Pour in the wine to deglaze the pan, turn up the heat and bring to the boil. Boil for 4–5 minutes, stirring until it reaches the consistency of syrup. Turn down the heat and add the barley, then put in about a third of the chicken stock, stirring all the time. Once it is starting to be absorbed, pour in the rest of the stock and cook until all is absorbed – about 35–40 minutes. Keep an eye on it and stir regularly. When the barleyotto is within 5–10 minutes of being cooked, stir in the chorizo and peppers, and grind over a good quantity of fresh black pepper, stirring in well. Take off the heat and stir in the basil. Serve with a sprinkle of basil sprigs and some fresh Parmesan shavings over the top.

There are more barleyotto recipes on page 92 and pages 154–5.

Goat's Cheese with Pear

Preparation time: 5 minutes, Serves 1

30g/½ cup goat's cheese
1 pear
Freshly ground black pepper

Slice the cheese and the pear, arrange on a plate and grind over the pepper – mmmm!

Greek-style Yoghurt with Nuts, Seeds, Mint and Fresh Ginger

Preparation time: 5 minutes, Serves 1

6 tbsp Toasted Seed Mix (see page 121)
250ml/1 cup Greek yoghurt (or natural bio yoghurt)
6 fresh mint leaves, torn
1 tsp grated fresh ginger

Stir all the ingredients together and drizzle with ½ tsp honey or fructose if needed. Lovely breakfast!

This is great with low-GL fruit as well.

Herby Cream Cheese

Preparation time: 7 minutes, Serves around 4

150g/½ cup half-fat cream cheese
150g/½ cup crème fraîche
1 tbsp of 5 of the following herbs (finely chopped): mint,
    chives, coriander (cilantro), parsley, marjoram, basil, thyme
    (depending on what is in season and your preference)
1 clove garlic, grated (optional)
Lots of freshly ground black pepper

Combine all the ingredients in a bowl (or blender). Delicious as a dip with crudités, oatcakes or a piece of hot low-GL toast.

Beef and Vegetable Casserole

Preparation time: 15 minutes, Cooking time: 1 hour, Serves 6

4 tbsp extra virgin olive oil

600g/5–6 cups good lean stewing steak, cubed

2 onions, sliced

4 cloves garlic, crushed or grated

2 courgettes (zucchini), cut into chunky rounds

2 tbsp white wine

600ml/2½ cups chicken or vegetable stock

2 carrots, cut into rounds

2 sticks celery, sliced

3 ripe tomatoes (or 1 small can tomatoes)

1 red pepper, cut into chunks

1-inch/3cm piece fresh ginger, grated finely (or ½ tsp
    powdered)

Plenty of freshly ground black pepper

Preheat the oven to 200°C/400°F/Gas Mark 6. Heat 2 tbsp of the olive oil in a large casserole dish (with a lid) over a medium-high hob. Fry the steak on each side to seal. Take out and put aside. Heat the remaining olive oil, add the onions and fry for a minute or two, being careful not to burn them. Put the steak back in, add the garlic and the courgettes and fry for a little longer. Deglaze the pan with the white wine (this is where the alcohol gets all the juicy cooking stuff off the bottom of the pan and makes sure those flavours are in the finished dish), and add the chicken or vegetable stock. Add the rest of the vegetables, grate in the ginger and bring to the boil. Put the lid on the dish and put in the oven.

Scrub 1 medium sweet potato per person and put in the oven to bake. Leave the casserole to cook for 45 minutes to an hour. Season to taste.

Pea and Mint Soup

Preparation time: 10 minutes, Cooking time: 20 minutes, Serves 4

1 tbsp extra virgin olive oil

1 onion, chopped finely

1 small or ½ large cauliflower, chopped

1 litre/4½ cups vegetable or chicken stock

450g petit pois/peas

Big handful fresh mint, chopped finely (reserve some for
    decoration)

Freshly ground black pepper

4 tbsp Greek-style natural yoghurt or crème fraîche

Heat the oil in a pan large enough to hold the soup. Add the onion and fry gently for a couple of minutes. Add the cauliflower and stock, bring to the boil and simmer for 10 minutes, then add the petit pois and mint. Season liberally. Simmer for another 5 minutes. Then liquidize, pour into bowls, swirl with the yoghurt, sprinkle with some mint, grind over some fresh black pepper and serve.

If you would like to add ham to this soup, choose a good quality ham, dice and add it just after the onion but before the cauliflower. This soup freezes well.

Scrambled Eggs with Smoked Salmon

Preparation time: 5 minutes, Cooking time: 5–7 minutes, Serves 2

Everyone has their own way of doing scrambled eggs – this is ours!

4 eggs
Small bunch chives, chopped finely (save some for garnish)
Freshly ground black pepper
1 tbsp butter
4 generous slices smoked salmon
1 lemon, cut into wedges

Beat the eggs in a bowl, then stir in the chives and black pepper. Melt the butter in a saucepan over a medium heat and add the eggs. Stir continuously until the eggs are cooked to your liking. Divide between two plates, drape with the smoked salmon, sprinkle over a few more chives, squeeze a lemon wedge over the top and grind over some black pepper. Delicious with a slice of low-GL toast.

Houmous

Preparation time: 10 minutes, Serves 4 as a dip

1 can (approx 410g/2 cups) chickpeas
2 tbsp tahini paste
2 cloves garlic, peeled
3 tbsp lemon juice
3 tbsp extra virgin olive oil
Couple of generous pinches of paprika
Sprinkling of chopped coriander (cilantro)

Put the chickpeas, tahini paste, garlic and lemon juice in a blender. As it blends, add about 3 tbsp of olive oil in a slow trickle. Taste the dip – it should be smooth and creamy. If it appears too dry, slowly drizzle in more oil. Sprinkle with paprika and some chopped coriander and a drizzle of olive oil. Serve with crudités or salad or a piece of hot low-GL toast.

Giant Prawns with Mucho-spicy Dip

Preparation time: 10 minutes, Chilling time: 1 hour,
Serves 8 as a dip, 4 as lunch/snack with salad

200g/1 cup/250ml crème fraîche/Greek-style yoghurt
1 tsp finely grated fresh root ginger (or generous pinch
    powdered ginger)
2 large cloves garlic, grated finely or crushed
1½ tsp grainy or Dijon mustard
1 tsp chopped fresh dill (or generous pinch dried dill)
1 tsp Worcester sauce

To serve
15–20 large peeled prawns
1 lemon, cut into wedges
Dill sprigs to garnish
Crispy salad (if having as a meal rather than a dip)

Mix all the ingredients together and put in the fridge to
chill for an hour or so. Put the dip in a nice bowl in the
middle of a plate/platter. Arrange the prawns around the
dip, garnish with lemon wedges and dill sprigs and serve.
Alternatively, serve with a crispy salad as a lunch/light
meal.

  What a great book. I saw the reasoning behind the popular GI diets but found it hard to put into practice. A book based on GL provided the missing link that helped me to make sense of this way of eating. At last a healthy 'diet' that didn't rely on gimmicks and left me feeling happy and satisfied. I'm now losing weight without feeling hungry or deprived, and as a bonus I have more energy and my skin glows with health. Thank you.

Mo G from Berkshire

Chapter 9

VARIETY IS THE SPICE OF LIFE

We hope you've enjoyed all the recipes in the seven-day plans. Here are some more, plus ideas for special occasions, a word on desserts, and guidance on how to adapt some of your favourite recipes to fit your low-GL lifestyle.

These are recipes for you to follow, play with, be inspired by and adapt to your own tastes. As in all the plans, you can leave out the garlic and chilli if you prefer, and use dried herbs for convenience.

A few of the recipes have been posted on our website by fabulous Diet Freedom Fighters. Visit our website for lots more recipes, as well as inspiration, help and support.

Happy cooking!

Chicken, Poultry and Other Meats

All these recipes work well with turkey, pork and other lean meats.

Andie's Greek Chicken

Preparation time: 20 minutes, Cooking time: 45 minutes, Serves 4

Andie is a real inspiration on the Diet Freedom forums – and we're very pleased she's shared this great recipe with us all. It's not one of the fastest, but it's really tasty – thanks Andie!

4 lemons, sliced thinly
4 bone-in chicken pieces with skin
8 cloves garlic, peeled
2 tbsp olive oil
1 tbsp fresh lemon juice
1 tbsp freshly ground black pepper
1 tbsp chopped fresh mint leaves
1 tbsp chopped fresh oregano
10 pitted kalamata olives, cut in half (optional)
100g feta cheese, crumbled

Arrange the shelf in the centre of the oven. Heat the oven to 180°C/350°F/Gas Mark 4. Layer lemon slices on the bottom of a large baking dish and set aside. Gently run your fingers between each chicken piece and the skin to loosen it. Press 2 garlic cloves through a garlic press. Lift the skin from one chicken piece and rub the garlic between skin and flesh. Repeat the process with the remaining chicken pieces and garlic cloves. Drizzle olive oil and lemon juice over the chicken. Sprinkle with pepper and rub into the skin. Place the chicken over the lemon slices in the prepared dish. Combine the mint and oregano in a small bowl; evenly sprinkle over the chicken breasts. Sprinkle olives over the chicken, if using. Bake for 45 minutes, until the juices run clear when the chicken is pricked with a fork. Remove from the oven and sprinkle with feta. Bake for 5 more minutes. Serve with pan juices and low-GL veggies or salad.

Chicken Breasts with Blue Cheese and Watercress

Preparation time: 10 minutes, Cooking time: 15–20 minutes, Serves 4

4 chicken breasts
2 tbsp olive oil
Freshly ground black pepper
160g/2 cups blue cheese (Stilton, dolcelatte, etc.)
1 medium bag fresh watercress

Cover the chicken in the olive oil and grind on plenty of black pepper. Put under a medium grill until almost cooked (about 10–15 minutes depending on the size of the chicken breasts – make sure the juice runs clear when you prick them). Remove the pan from under the grill. Divide the cheese into four and crumble on top of the chicken breasts, then grill the chicken again until the cheese has melted.

Divide the watercress between four plates. Put each chicken breast on the watercress. Serve with a tomato salad dressed with olive oil and balsamic vinegar or low-GL vegetables.

Spicy Peanut Chicken

Preparation time: 10 minutes, Cooking time: 15–20 minutes, Serves 4

50g/½ cup peanuts
1 tsp ground mixed spice
½–1 tsp chilli powder (depending on how hot you like it)
4 chicken breasts
1 free range egg, beaten

Grind the peanuts in a blender and mix in the spices. Put the mixture on a plate. Dip the chicken breasts in the egg, then in the peanut mix. Grill or bake until cooked thoroughly. Serve with low-GL veggies or salad.

Variations
- This also makes a good kebab recipe for the barbecue.
- For a 'warm chicken salad', cook the chicken as above, slice and toss into a salad of lovely leaves. Dress with lemon juice and olive oil and plenty of black pepper.

Soups

Soup is much underrated and is a great standby.

Tomato, Garlic and Basil Soup

Preparation time: 10 minutes, Cooking time: 10 minutes, Serves 2

2 cans (approximately 800g/4 cups) tomatoes in juice
4 cloves garlic
1 tsp freshly ground black pepper
1 tsp chilli flakes
1 tsp paprika or smoked paprika
1 tsp crushed cardamom seeds
2 big handfuls basil (or 2 tbsp pesto)
250ml/1 cup water or chicken stock
1 tablespoon Greek yoghurt/half-fat crème fraîche

Throw all the ingredients into a blender and whiz. Pour into a pan and heat. Remove from the heat and stir in the yoghurt or crème fraîche. Serve with a piece of low-GL toast, another dollop of yoghurt or crème fraîche and a few basil leaves for colour.

Variations
- Add a bit of fresh grated ginger for some extra zing.
- Use chicken stock rather than water.

Fish

Spicy Chilli Prawns

Preparation time: 5 minutes, Marinating time: 30 minutes, Cooking time: 5 minutes, Serves 4 with salad

2 cloves garlic, crushed or grated

3 tbsp olive or avocado oil

1 small fresh red chilli, deseeded and chopped finely (or ½ tsp hot chilli flakes)

10–15 large peeled prawns, or 225g smaller ones

2 tbsp chopped coriander (cilantro)

To serve

Crisp salad

1 lemon, cut into wedges

Coriander sprigs

Place all ingredients (except the coriander) in a large bowl and marinate the prawns for about 30 minutes. Fry the prawns in their marinade on a medium-high heat for 2–3 minutes. Remove from the heat and stir in the chopped coriander. Serve with a crisp salad, and garnish with lemon wedges and coriander sprigs.

Haddock with Spinach, Mushrooms and Crème Fraîche

Preparation time: 10 minutes, Cooking time: 20–30 minutes, Serves 2

This recipe was posted on our website by Caroline, who originally suggested it as a dish using chicken breasts (which works very well). Jo then tried it with haddock and recommended it highly too, so here we have a combination of inspiration from them both!

2 fresh haddock fillets
1 bag fresh spinach leaves
100g/1½ cups mushrooms, sliced
1 tsp English mustard
5 tbsp crème fraîche
Handful of fresh tarragon
150g/3 cups half-fat Cheddar, grated
Plenty of freshly ground black pepper

Preheat the oven to 200°C/400°F/Gas Mark 6. Place the haddock fillets in a lightly oiled baking tin, cover with the fresh spinach, then the sliced mushrooms. Mix the mustard into a small pot of crème fraîche and pour over. Sprinkle with the tarragon, top with the grated cheese and season with freshly ground black pepper. Bake for 20–30 minutes and serve with your choice of veggies. Caroline recommends cauliflower and carrot mash, broccoli and peas.

Grilled Mackerel and Cheese on Toast

Preparation time: 5 minutes, Cooking time: 3 minutes, Serves 2

This is a great snack. It comes from Joanne, who swears by it as a swift lunch or snack on oatcakes.

1 tin mackerel
1 spring onion, chopped finely
Plenty of freshly ground black pepper
2 pieces low-GL toast
Juice of ½ a lemon
Thin slices of any cheese to put on top
Dash of Worcester sauce

Preheat the grill to high. Mash the mackerel, spring onion and black pepper together and spread on the toast. Squeeze over some lemon juice. Put a very thin layer of cheese on top, sprinkle with a little Worcester sauce and grill until bubbling. Serve at once with a crisp salad.

Variation
Deborah goes on about sprouted beans, as we know! They are great on toast with a thin layer of cheese on top like this, and grilled hot and fast – really delicious and fresh-tasting.

'Barleyotto'

Pearl barley is an excellent substitute for rice in risotto-style dishes. And to expand on our previous recipes (see Chapters 7 and 8), here are some fantastic variations.

The basic barleyotto recipe to serve 4–6 as follows:

25g/2 tbsp butter or olive oil-based spread

1 tsp olive oil

1 medium onion or 3 shallots, diced

2–3 cloves garlic, grated or crushed

100ml/½ cup dry white wine

200g/1 cup pearl barley

700ml/3 cups chicken stock

Melt the butter or spread and the olive oil in a large pan over a medium heat. Add the onion and, stirring gently, fry for about a minute. Add the garlic and cook for just 1 more minute, taking care not to let the garlic burn. Pour in the wine to deglaze the pan, turn up the heat and bring to the boil. Boil for 4–5 minutes, stirring until it reaches the consistency of syrup. Turn down the heat and add the barley, then put in about a third of the chicken stock, stirring all the time. Once it is starting to be absorbed, pour in the rest of the stock, and cook until it has all been absorbed, about 35–40 minutes. Keep an eye on it and stir regularly.

Variations

Prawn, Asparagus and Pea Barleyotto

Five minutes before your barleyotto is cooked, add 4 cups of large prawns, 3 cups of peas and about 12 asparagus tips (when in season), stirring in to ensure all are warmed through and lightly cooked. Serve sprinkled with mint leaves and Parmesan shavings.

Lemon, Chicken and Herb Barleyotto

Handful fresh mint
1 sprig fresh rosemary
1 sprig fresh sage
Zest of 1 lemon
Olive oil
4 chicken breasts, cut into strips
15g (1 tbsp) butter
Juice of ½ lemon

De-sprig and chop all the herbs finely together, mix with the lemon zest and set aside. Cook the chicken in a little olive oil in a large saucepan as your barleyotto is cooking. Sear on quite a high heat to begin with and then cook until the meat runs clear when poked with a knife. Remove from the heat and set aside. Once the barleyotto is cooked, stir in the chicken, herbs and butter, and squeeze the lemon juice over. Serve immediately, sprinkled with a few herbs.

Perfect Pasta

It's a myth that you can't eat pasta on a low-GL diet. Here are a few ways to mitigate the high-GL of pasta with delicious low-GL ingredients.

- Keep all pasta portions to around 100g cooked weight per person.
- Fresh pasta filled with meat, spinach or cheese will have a lower GL than unfilled pasta. However, filled pasta is often quite high in fat.
- Egg fettuccine is one of the lowest-GL pastas, and wholemeal pasta is slightly lower than white.
- Boil pasta only until *al dente* or just cooked.
- Serve pasta in a sauce as a side dish with other vegetables, beans and pulses.
- Many gluten-free pastas have an even higher GL than wheat pasta. Your best alternatives are vegetable pastas or pasta made with buckwheat or spelt. Although neither buckwheat nor spelt pasta has been formally tested for its GL score, we are making an educated guess that they will be on a par or lower than the refined wheat pastas because they are usually made from stoneground flour.
- Homemade vegetable pasta is great! Cut any of your favourite veg into strips, steam or blanch them for a few seconds, then drain and use as pasta with your favourite sauces.

Minty Yoghurt, Sugar Snap and Sun-dried Tomato Pasta Sauce

Preparation time: 5 minutes, Cooking time: 5 minutes plus pasta cooking time, Serves 4 people (100g cooked weight of pasta for anyone following the GL plan)

200g sugar snap peas (or mangetout), topped and tailed
500ml/2 cups Greek-style yoghurt (or other natural yoghurt)
Juice of ½ lemon
Zest of 1 lemon
2 tbsp olive oil
10 sun-dried tomatoes, chopped roughly into strips
Small handful chopped fresh mint (about 3 tbsp once
    chopped)
4 tbsp Parmesan cheese, grated
Freshly grated black pepper, to serve

Boil the pasta as per instructions on the packet. About 2 minutes before the pasta is cooked *al dente*, add the sugar snaps. Drain the pasta and sugar snaps, and return to the pan. Mix the yoghurt with the lemon juice and zest until blended and not separated. Add the olive oil to the pasta and toss, then add the sun-dried tomatoes, mint, Parmesan and yoghurt mix. Toss together with plenty of freshly ground black pepper and serve immediately.

Keeping it Simple

For a quick meal, we also like pasta cooked *al dente* then tossed with:

- Roughly chopped artichoke hearts in their oil, some Parmesan, and freshly ground black pepper.
- Pesto, sun-dried tomatoes (use some of the oil they come in too) and Parmesan with lots of fresh black pepper.
- Chopped peppers from a jar, 1 clove grated garlic, olive oil and plenty of black pepper – this is great if you throw the ingredients in the pan the pasta has been cooked in while it is draining in the sieve in the sink. Cook for literally a minute to warm through then add the pasta, stir through and serve.
- Chopped ham, sun-dried tomatoes, basil, olive oil, black pepper.
- Bought sauces as per the food lists (see Chapter 10).

If you don't overdo the pasta portions and serve it with plenty of lovely crisp salad or some other low-GL veggies, you will have a lowish-GL meal.

Salads

Salad is truly fabulous. And this from three folk who used to think leaves were for rabbits, fitness freaks or dreary draconian diets! We're total converts now and we hope the following recipes will get you into the salad-loving habit too. You know you want to … grab some of your favourite leaves and dress them up!

Warm French Bean Salad

Preparation and cooking time: 10 minutes, Serves 4 as a side dish

400g/4 generous handfuls green beans, topped and tailed
1 red chilli, deseeded and diced
1 tbsp light soy sauce
½ tbsp toasted sesame oil
3 tbsp sesame seeds

Boil or steam the beans until tender yet still crisp. Meanwhile, mix the other ingredients together. Toss the beans in the mix, and serve as a side dish.

Bacon, Quinoa and Rocket Salad with Warm Dressing

Preparation and cooking time: 20 minutes, Serves 6 as a starter, 4 as a main course

4 tbsp extra virgin olive oil

250g/2 cups roughly chopped lean bacon

2 cloves garlic

Pinch of paprika

120g/½ cup quinoa (around 30g per person as a main course)

Generous handful of rocket and watercress leaves (or mix of
    your favourite leaves) per person

1 tbsp balsamic vinegar

Juice of ½ a lemon

Freshly ground black pepper, to serve

4 spring onions, chopped

Heat the oil in a large frying pan over a medium-high heat and fry the bacon. Once golden, turn the heat down and add the garlic and paprika.

Bring 1 litre/4½ cups of water to the boil in a pan. Rinse the quinoa under warm water in a sieve then put it in the boiling water and cook on a fast simmer for 12–15 minutes. Drain and set aside.

Arrange the salad leaves in a large bowl (or on individual plates if you prefer). Remove the bacon pan from the heat. Stir in the quinoa, vinegar, lemon juice and black pepper. Pour over the salad, scatter with spring onions, toss and serve immediately.

Variation
Bulgur wheat or amaranth would also work well in this salad in place of quinoa – cook as per packet instructions and incorporate as above.

Bacon and Bean Salad

**Preparation time: 10 minutes, Cooking time: 20 minutes,
Serves 4 as a starter or side salad**

1 tsp caraway seeds

½ tsp cumin seeds, crushed (or pinch of ground cumin)

4 tbsp extra virgin olive oil

1 large red onion, chopped (not too finely)

6 slices smoked bacon

2–4 cloves garlic, grated or crushed

820g/4 cups haricot beans (usually come in 410g tins),
   drained and rinsed (mixing a tin of butter beans and a tin of
   haricot beans together also gives a great result, and
   chickpeas are another good alternative)

Freshly ground black pepper

Handful of fresh herbs (basil, parsley, mint, etc.),
   chopped/ripped roughly

Heat a large dry frying pan over a medium-high heat. Put the caraway seeds and cumin into the pan, and move the pan about for about 30 seconds or until you can smell the spice aroma. Then add the olive oil and the onion and allow to sweat on the same heat – without burning – for a couple of minutes. Add in the bacon, garlic and the beans and plenty of black pepper. Stir until everything is coated in oil, turn down to a medium heat and cook, stirring occasionally, for about 15–20 minutes. Remove from the heat, stir in the fresh herbs and serve as a side dish. If you would like this cold, perhaps for a lunch-box snack, then allow to cool, then add some chopped cherry tomatoes, maybe some lemon juice and a little more oil, and the herbs.

Melon and Mint with Halloumi Cheese

Preparation time: 10 minutes, Cooking time: 5 minutes, Serves 2

1 tbsp extra virgin olive oil

½ tbsp caraway seeds (optional)

1 packet halloumi cheese, cut into thick chunks (about
1cm/½ inch)

2 large slices of your favourite melon, or a mixture of types,
cut into chunks

Generous handful of mint, chopped roughly

Heat a frying pan over a medium-high heat with the olive oil and caraway seeds. Add the halloumi cheese and allow to fry until golden brown on both sides. Put the melon chunks into a large bowl, add the mint and toss. Pour over the halloumi when cooked, adding any oil from the pan, and toss. Serve immediately.

Variations

This is a great lunch-box salad if you use feta cheese, pecorino (Italian ewe's cheese), or Edam.

Sumptuous Salad Dressings and Marinades

Warm Toasted Sesame Dressing

Preparation time: 7 minutes

1 tbsp sesame seeds

2 tbsp sesame oil (or toasted sesame oil for extra 'toastiness'!)

4 tbsp extra virgin olive oil

Light grating of nutmeg (equivalent to a 'pinch')

1 tbsp light vinegar (not dark, use white wine vinegar or
    similar)

Place the sesame seeds in a dry frying pan and toast on a warm hob until they start to turn golden. Turn the heat down to medium, add the oils and the nutmeg and allow to warm and infuse for about 3–5 minutes. Turn off the heat, pour in the vinegar and allow to warm through – another minute at the most. Pour into a jug, whisk and pour. If you prefer it cold, don't add the vinegar to the pan – pour it all into a jug and allow to cool.

Creamy Olive Tapenade Dressing

Preparation time: 7 minutes

100g/1 cup pitted black (or green, or a mix) olives
8–10 anchovy fillets, drained
1 tbsp capers, drained
4 tbsp extra virgin olive oil
Zest and juice of 1 lemon
½ tsp grainy mustard
250ml/1 cup crème fraîche or natural yoghurt

Place everything except the crème fraîche in a blender and blend into a rough paste. Put into a bowl and stir in the crème fraîche.

This is fabulous with fish or roasted veg, or as an alternative 'Caesar' dressing when using tuna in the salad. If you'd like a runnier dressing, use a thinner yoghurt or stir in up to 4 tablespoons of water.

Herby Oils and Vinegars

Oils and vinegars that are full of herbs and spices make the fastest, easiest dressings and marinades (for more about oils, see Chapter 12). Always check the label to make sure the herbs and spices are the only additives!

You can make your own infused oils and vinegars by adding your favourite herbs and spices. Don't get hung up on the amounts or specific blends. For example, if you have a handful of fresh basil left over and a handy bottle of white wine vinegar, stuff the basil in the bottle and let it infuse for a week or so. Yum! Or use the suggested combinations below:

- Chilli (fresh, whole or in flakes), garlic and black pepper
- Rosemary (thoroughly washed and dried) and garlic
- Lemongrass and coriander (cilantro)
- Basil (bash it a bit first), garlic and sun-dried tomatoes

Don't let this put you off the classic oil and vinegar combination, or the lemon juice and vinegar alternative. And if you're hankering for the exotic, make a simple but gorgeous dressing by cutting a pomegranate in half and squeezing it over your salad – seeds and all.

All-round Blend for Marinades and Dressings

3 sprigs rosemary

8 sprigs thyme

3 large cloves, cut into 3

3–5 small hot red chilli peppers

6 cardamom pods (bash a bit so they split)

6–8 juniper berries

10 capers, drained (the best ones are in brine)

Pour oil or vinegar into a clean bottle or jar. Add the washed and dried herbs and spices and let it steep for a week. Keep cool and use within a couple of weeks.

These also make great gifts but worry not – we're not about to get all arts and crafts on you!

Veggie Mashes

All these mash recipes, and variations thereof, make fantastic toppings for shepherd's pie, cottage pie and fish pie.

Creamy Cauliflower Mash with Grainy Mustard and Parmesan

Preparation time: 5 minutes, Cooking time: 10 minutes, Serves 6 as a side dish

1 large cauliflower, cut into chunks (around 8 pieces)
2 tbsp grainy mustard
2 tbsp crème fraîche/natural Greek-style yoghurt
80g grated Parmesan, mature Cheddar or other strong-tasting cheese
Freshly ground black pepper, to taste

Boil or steam the cauliflower and drain well (if you don't it will be too watery). Put back into the saucepan and mash – unlike potato it doesn't need to be really smooth. Then stir in the rest of the ingredients.

Celeriac Mash with Spring Onions and Chives

Preparation time: 5 minutes, Cooking time: 15 minutes, Serves 6 as a side dish

1 medium celeriac, peeled and cut into chunks
2 tbsp butter or crème fraîche
Freshly ground black pepper, to taste
4 tbsp chives, chopped
2 spring onions, chopped

Boil or steam the celeriac until cooked. Drain well, put back in the pan and mash. Stir in the rest of the ingredients and season well.

Carrot and Coriander Mash

Preparation time: 5 minutes, Cooking time: 15–20 minutes,
Serves 6 as a side dish

Inspired by the fabulous soup, here's a twist!

500g carrots, peeled and chopped
3 cloves garlic, chopped roughly
2 tbsp butter or olive oil-based spread
Freshly ground black pepper, to taste
1 large bunch coriander (cilantro), chopped quite finely

Boil or steam the carrots with the garlic until tender. Drain, put back into the pan, mash with the butter and plenty of black pepper. Stir in the coriander. Serve immediately.

Veggie Side Dishes

Zingy New Potatoes

**Preparation time: 6 minutes, Cooking time: 10–12 minutes,
Serves 6 as a side dish**

It's a myth that you can't eat any potatoes on a low-GL
diet. Cook them lightly and eat them as a side dish rather
than as part of the main course. Enjoy!

500g new potatoes
Handful of parsley and any other fresh herb you like
3 tbsp extra virgin olive oil
2 tbsp balsamic vinegar
Juice of ½ a lemon
1 tsp red peppercorns

Cut the potatoes in half and boil for 8–12 minutes or until
tender (prod with a skewer or knife – if it goes in smoothly
and comes out quickly then the potato is done). Drain
and put in a bowl. Chop the herbs and scatter over the
potatoes. Mix together the olive oil, balsamic vinegar and
lemon juice and pour over the potatoes. Crush the
peppercorns and sprinkle over, then toss and serve with
other low-GL veggies.

Chilli, Lime and Garlic Spinach

Preparation time: 5 minutes, Cooking time: 15–20 minutes,
Serves 2 as a side dish

This recipe comes from another Diet Freedom Fighter, Lesley Hutchinson, and in her own words: 'Trying to find an exciting way to liven up spinach, I experimented and came up with a deliciously low-GL recipe which is so healthy you can eat it till it comes out of your ears. Don't breathe on anyone afterwards though! It would probably work pretty well with other veg too.'

1 bag fresh, blanched spinach (or ½ bag frozen spinach, defrosted)
2 tbsp olive oil
1 fresh red chilli, deseeded and chopped (or 1 tsp chilli flakes or powder)
5 cloves garlic, grated or crushed
3 tbsp soy sauce
Zest and juice of 1 lime

Preheat the oven to 220°C/425°F/Gas Mark 7. Drain the spinach and put into an ovenproof dish with the olive oil, fresh chilli and garlic and soy sauce. Squeeze in some lime juice and a little zest too. Cook for around 15–20 minutes.

There is another great spinach recipe on our website – Fran's Fabulous Spanish Spinach. We're very keen that wonderful, healthy greens get a makeover and become a more regular part of everyone's diet.

Roasted Tomatoes

**Preparation time: 10 minutes, Cooking time: 40 minutes,
Serves 4 as a side dish**

8 big ripe tomatoes (or 4 beef tomatoes)
8 cloves garlic, unpeeled
3 bay leaves
4 tbsp olive oil
1 tsp dried oregano
1 tsp dried thyme
1 tbsp sesame seeds
Freshly ground black pepper

Preheat the oven to 220°C/425°F/Gas Mark 7. Wash and
dry the tomatoes and place closely packed in a baking tin.
Push the garlic cloves and bay leaves between them, pour
over the olive oil and sprinkle with the herbs, sesame
seeds and black pepper. Bake for around 40 minutes.
Serve as a side dish with the juices.

Baking and Desserts

We all know that cakes, biscuits and desserts are likely to slow down any weight loss – let's be honest. However, over at Diet Freedom HQ we're working very hard to forage for treats that are delicious, low-GL *and* healthy. It is possible, and there are some really interesting new ideas coming out – including our own range of Diet Freedom healthy treats.

In the meantime, here are a few indulgent and healthy desserts you can use as treats.

Apricot 'Jam'

Preparation time: 10 minutes, Cooking time: 10 minutes

This is not jam as such, but makes a really good jam substitute on low-GL bread. You could add a spoonful to yoghurt or use it in baking. It will keep for a few days in the fridge.

200g dried apricots (organic where possible)
60ml water
1 tbsp fructose

Place the apricots in a small saucepan with the water, bring to the boil and simmer quickly for about 5 minutes – keep the apricots under water where possible, and be really careful not to let it boil dry. Take off the heat and stir in the fructose. Let it cool a bit and then liquidize. Put in a sealed container and keep in the fridge.

Blackberry and Apple Crumble

Preparation time: 15 minutes, Cooking time: 30 minutes, Serves 4

3 large cooking apples

4 tbsp water

2 tbsp fructose

1 tsp cinnamon powder

1 cup/2 handfuls blackberries (you can use other fruit too)

225g/1 cup porridge oats

50g/¾ cup ground almonds

1 tbsp butter or olive oil-based spread

Preheat the oven to 180°C/350°F/Gas Mark 4. Peel, core and slice the apples, and put in a saucepan with the water. Put the pan over a medium heat and cook the apples for about 10 minutes or until they have softened. Stir in 1 tablespoon of the fructose and the cinnamon, and let it cook gently for another few minutes. Remove from the heat and stir in the blackberries. Transfer to an ovenproof baking dish and set aside.

In a mixing bowl combine the oats, almonds and remaining fructose, then rub in the butter or spread with your fingers until you have a crumbly mixture. Pour this evenly over the fruit in the baking dish. Put this in the oven and bake for about 20–30 minutes – the fruit doesn't need much cooking, but you want a nice brown topping! Serve warm with Greek-style natural yoghurt, crème fraîche or a spoonful of cream.

Variations
You can add desiccated coconut to the crumble topping, as well as a combination of seeds.

Strawberry and Fresh Fig Brûlée

Preparation time: 15 minutes, Serves 4

4 ripe fresh figs, sliced
8 fresh strawberries, halved
1 vanilla pod (or 1 tsp vanilla essence)
150ml/¼ pint double (heavy) cream
150ml/¼ pint crème fraîche
4 egg yolks
1 tsp fructose
2 tsp fructose, for sprinkling

Place the fruit into and around the edges of 4 large ramekin dishes. Place the vanilla pod in a pan. Stir in the two creams and heat to just below boiling point. Remove the pod. Beat the egg yolks and fructose together in a pan, then gradually beat in the hot vanilla cream. Heat gently until the sauce has thickened. Pour the custard over the fruit in the ramekins and set aside to cool. When cool, chill for 2–3 hours until set. Sprinkle the puddings with a little fructose and place under a preheated hot grill to form a caramelized coating. Serve cold.

Variation
You can change the fruits to any low-GL ones you prefer.

Yoghurts

You can simply combine your low-GL fruit and yoghurt. We've put together a couple of yoghurt variations to keep your taste buds interested! The measurements don't need to be as precise as in the recipes. They're intended just to give you guidelines and inspiration.

Vanilla and Blueberry Yoghurt

Preparation time: 5 minutes, Serves 2

250ml/1 cup natural bio yoghurt (or ½ bio/½ Greek-style, or ½
   crème fraîche/½ bio)
50g/½ cup blueberries
½ tsp vanilla essence
1 tsp fructose

Mix and serve immediately or store in the fridge – will last a couple of days.

Variations
Any low-GL fruit will work. However, berries or bananas are particularly good. If you want a smooth yoghurt, then blend the ingredients together in a liquidizer.

Banana, Mint and Raspberry Yoghurt with Toasted Seeds

Preparation time: 5 minutes, Serves 2

250ml/1 cup natural bio yoghurt (or ½ bio/½ Greek-style, or ½
    crème fraîche/½ bio)
1 medium banana (80–100g without skin, not too ripe as per
    food lists in Chapter 10)
Generous handful of mint leaves
50g/¾ cup raspberries

To serve
4 tbsp toasted seeds (page 121) or just dry-toast your
    favourite seed mix in a frying pan over a medium heat)
Mint sprigs

Put the yoghurt, banana and mint in a blender and whizz
until fully mixed. Transfer to a bowl and mix in the raspberries. Divide into individual bowls and sprinkle with the
toasted seeds and mint sprigs. If you're not serving it
immediately, put it in the fridge and keep the seeds separate to sprinkle on before serving – they tend to go a bit
soggy otherwise.

Special Occasions

The Sunday roast lunch (on whichever day you do it) is the perfect low-GL feast. Tips to follow are:

- Stick to lean roast cuts and good-quality free-range poultry for the overall health factor.
- Roast a selection of veggies – celeriac, carrots, a parsnip, butternut squash, other squashes, onions, garlic, a few new potatoes.
- Serve with fresh steamed veggies – peas, broccoli, cabbage, etc., or some mash – sweet potato, cauliflower or butter bean.

You'll find a number of veggie side dishes in this chapter, all of which make a great accompaniment to a Sunday roast.

Perhaps our favourite roast is chicken, so here's a recipe.

Drunken Gin and Juniper Roast Chicken

Preparation time: 10 minutes, Cooking time: 1–1½ hours, Serves 6

1 medium whole roasting chicken

1 bulb garlic, broken into cloves and bashed (no need to peel, just make sure the skin is pierced so the flavour gets out)

2 lemons, quartered

10 dried juniper berries, crushed (if you can't find them in the spice rack then just add an extra slug of gin – purely for the flavour, of course)

4 sprigs rosemary

1 onion, quartered

4 tbsp olive oil

Plenty of freshly ground black pepper

1 tsp allspice, ground

4 tbsp gin

4 cups water

Preheat the oven to 180°C/350°F/Gas Mark 4. To prepare the chicken, bash 6 cloves of garlic and put these and 4 lemon wedges into the cavity of the chicken along with half of the juniper berries. Put the rosemary in the bottom of a large roasting tin, and put the chicken on top. Scatter the remainder of the juniper berries, the garlic cloves and the onion around the chicken. Pour the olive oil over the top of the chicken, grind lots of pepper and sprinkle with allspice, and rub into the skin. Then pour the gin over the chicken, and pour the water into the roasting tin. Cover the tin with foil so it is as airtight as possible (if you've got a chicken brick or a big enough casserole then use that), and cook for the first hour. Then remove the foil, check on the progress of the chicken, and put back so the skin browns a little more and it is thoroughly cooked through. Serve with some of the lovely low-GL veggie side dishes from earlier in the chapter – roasted veg or mash.

Outrageously Indulgent Celebration Cake

Preparation time: 30 minutes, Cooking time: 35–40 minutes, Cooling and icing time: 1½ hours

There are a few stages on the road to perfection with this incredibly indulgent, *special occasion only*, rich and delicious chocolate cake. So set the time aside and you will be amply rewarded with ummmms and aaaaaahs and cries of disbelief if you let on it is still comparatively low-GL! We love Joanne for helping us create this.

Because measurements are important with this cake we have not used cups, only grams.

For the cake

110g chocolate – 70% cocoa solids or more

85g butter

80g fructose

3 eggs, separated

2 tbsp ground almonds

For the icing

110g chocolate – 70% cocoa solids or more

110ml double (heavy) cream

Preheat the oven to 180°C/350°F/Gas Mark 4. Line and grease a 10cm/4-inch round cake mould (this makes a tall fluffy cake; you can use a bigger tin, but you might not get as much gooeyness in the middle). Melt the chocolate in a bowl over a pan of hot water. Once it's completely melted, mix in the butter and, once that's melted in, stir in the fructose. Take off the heat. Beat the egg yolks and stir them into the chocolate mixture. Whisk the egg whites until quite stiff. With a metal spoon, fold one spoonful of the egg whites into the chocolate mixture to 'slacken' it. Then gently fold in the rest of the egg whites. Pour into the cake tin, put into the oven and bake for about 35 minutes. It should still be slightly gooey in the middle. It will sink a bit when it comes out of the oven so don't be alarmed. Let it cool for a few minutes in the tin and then turn it out and let it cool completely on a wire rack.

To make the icing, put the chocolate in a bowl over a pan of hot water on the hob, add the cream and gently heat until the chocolate is melted. Stir the mixture together and set aside until the cake is completely cool. You might want to slice off the top of the cake so it is even, and then ice it with the chocolate and cream icing. Let it cool completely, and then put in the fridge overnight. Serve small pieces – it's incredibly rich!

Other Inspirations!

Easy Herbs

When you have too many fresh herbs left over – either from the garden in the summer, or when you've bought them for a particular dish – just stick them in a bag in the freezer and bingo: fresh non-maintenance herbs on demand. Or if they are chopped, sprinkle them into an ice-cube tray, fill it with water, freeze and use as needed.

Herb Butter

Melt some butter and chop herbs finely. Stir the herbs into the melted butter, pour into an ice-cube tray and freeze. Each herby butter cube will give you around 20g butter, which is about 1 $\frac{1}{2}$ tbsp.

Herby Vinegar

Make sure the herbs are clean, bug-free and dry! Put into a clean bottle and cover with white wine (or similar light) vinegar. If you have an open bottle of vinegar and a handful of leftover herbs the whole process takes minutes, and once you let the flavours steep together you'll have a tasty vinegar.

Making Your Favourite Recipes Low-GL

We would suggest holding back on the wild dessert and baking experiments until you've done the weight-loss bit and are maintaining your new and fabulous figure with ease. Nut flours and most desserts (like the outrageous cake on page 184) are still very calorie dense, and whilst calories are not top priority in the GL world, they are still relevant.

Baking

If you want to experiment with baking then nut flours are a good low-GL substitute. However, as they don't contain gluten they don't rise as well as normal flours. You won't get big fluffy loaves of bread or high-rise sponge cakes, but you can get some really nice results that taste delicious.

You can make great cheesecake bases with ground almonds and other nuts, a little butter or olive oil-based spread and a tablespoon of fructose instead of crushed biscuits – very tasty. There is a crumble recipe on page 104 – this, with a little more fat, would also make a good base.

There is a tasty bread recipe on page 116. If you've got a bread machine then take a look at the recipes in the booklet that came with it and see where you can adapt. For example, in wholewheat recipes that include strong white flour, you might want to substitute spelt or rye flour for the white. Adding a few tablespoons of linseeds/flax seeds or crushed nuts and sesame seeds will lower the GL and add interesting flavour to the bread.

As long as you make sure the weight of the dry ingredients – specifically the flour – is the same as in the recipe, you should get some good results. It may be that you add in some oats, oat bran, rye flakes and maybe some rye or spelt flour to the scales first, and then make up the dry flour weight with flour. As we've said before, you won't get the airy, almost tasteless, fluffy bread that comes from highly processed white flour, but you will get some really interesting wholesome darker breads and no blood sugar roller coaster. Hurrah!

You can make a sponge cake perfectly well with 100-per-cent wholemeal flour and almond flour (half and half perhaps), and use a third less fructose than the sugar amount stipulated in the recipe. Bear in mind that fructose browns more than sugar at higher oven temperatures.

Gram flour and nut flours are good in savoury recipes. If you want to thicken gravy or sauces then a spoonful of cornflour (cornstarch) in an otherwise low-GL meal will not be a problem. If you would like to try alternatives, however, you can use xantham gum or ground arrowroot, both of which are in many supermarkets and health-food shops.

Buckwheat pancakes are delicious, especially with freshly squeezed lemon and a little fructose. Go with your usual pancake recipe or look for a 'buckwheat galette' recipe – it's a very French thing. Play with savoury fillings as well, and serve with interesting salad combos.

Once you get used to bypassing high-GL, highly refined and processed ingredients it really becomes a great journey of exploration and taste – we promise!

PART IV

LIVING A LOW-GL LIFESTYLE

This part of the book is full of essential information to help make food choices and shopping as easy as possible. It contains an up-to-date list of low-GL foods in an easy, clear format, as well as a guide to stress-free shopping. Remember to use these lists as 'guides' – don't fall into the trap of treating them like a list of stringent 'rules'. The 7-day GL diet is a very easy way of life – not a military campaign!

You'll find:

- A list of foods with their GL ratings and portion guidelines.
- A shopping guide giving you the lowdown on what's hot and what's not – from supermarkets to farmers' markets.
- A whistle-stop tour of eating out GL style.
- A guide to healthy eating – love your food *and* your body!

66 The GL plan was a breath of fresh air. For years I had struggled with weight loss, even when I exercised regularly and ate regular 'low-fat' snacks and meals (like wholemeal toast and rice cakes with jacket potato at lunch). I would work hard and eat healthily but my weight loss always seemed to plateau. I ate larger quantities because low-fat food never left me full or satisfied. I also had very bad PMS-related food cravings, and basically would lose weight for 20 days a month only to put it back during the other 10 days. Then I'd get frustrated and think 'Why bother?'

Reading the GL plan I realized I probably had the wrong balance – too much starch (which was turning into sugar) and not enough fresh vegetables. The emphasis on natural, unprocessed food with the option of limited oil or cream made my meals tasty and satisfying. I was happy to load my plate up with veg, some of the wonderful sauces and main meals, and didn't miss the bread or potatoes. I used the recipes and, most importantly, viewed the process as a way of eating and ordering out at restaurants rather than as a 'diet'. My food cravings lessened and, together with regular exercise, I managed to bust through my personal weight-loss plateau to go from a size 18 to a 14 and to get below 12 stone and on to my lowest adult weight after literally years of trying. 99

Helga H from Birmingham

Chapter 10

LOW-GL FOOD LISTS WITH PORTION GUIDE

The following list of foods has been devised to guide you towards a healthier, lower-GL diet. We aren't going to tell you the GL of a doughnut, for instance, as we don't really want to encourage you to eat one! So let's stick with good, nutritious foods and lower-GL snacks and treats – no sugar rush equals no cravings!

For those of you who like numbers, we have included portion sizes to give you a GL of 10 or less. Foods listed as 10 GL or under are low-GL. However, as most of us hate weighing and measuring, that's all it is – an at-a-glance guide for those of us who need that extra bit of comfort. As we have said before, we are all very different – hence the three different food plans. As far as food quantities are concerned, for an easy, laid-back approach you can use the 'eat no more food than you can fit into your cupped hands at each meal' guideline; or for those who are less confident, you can use the portion guidelines as listed. Either way, remember to eat until you are satisfied and not stuffed!

Some foods are so low in available carbohydrates per serving that they are impossible to test for their GL – most berries for example. Foods that are normally made up of less than five per cent carbohydrate have a minimal impact on your blood sugar levels. These foods are included in the lists but we have marked 0 in the GL column for them. 'NT' in the GL column means that the food hasn't been tested yet. We have included such foods because they are nutritious and we assume they have a lowish GL.

As GI/GL testing is ongoing, we aim to give you the most up-to-date information available. Any foods tested after the publication of this book will be listed on our website.

We are all different (very boring indeed if we weren't) and so the amount of food we can eat while losing weight depends on a number of factors. These include our age, gender, activity level, metabolic rate and genetics to some degree. But lowering the overall GL of our diet by using the guidelines below will help keep blood sugar levels balanced and provide a constant, steady supply of energy from *slow* carbs, thus avoiding the highs and lows that can have us all wanting to nod off mid-afternoon after a high-GL lunch!

The following 'main' food list has been grouped into 'types' of food and has some extra notes and information. You will also find a condensed alphabetical list in Appendix 1 (without extra notes). Do read the notes and guidance on this list first, though, as you should find them helpful as you start your new way of eating.

PLEASE NOTE: All portions are cooked weights (if the food would normally be eaten cooked) unless otherwise stated.

BREAKFAST CEREALS

	Average portion	GL	Notes
Bran sticks	30g	NT	Not tested but has no added sugar so should have a fairly low GL – available from health-food stores.
Muesli	30g	7–16	Contents vary significantly as does the GL. Toasted has a lower GL. Always choose sugar-free versions, or use the recipe on page 112.
Porridge oats (steel cut cooked in water)	30g (dry weight)	9	A great low-GL choice for breakfast with chopped low-GL fresh fruit – see list on page 199.

MEAT

Choose fresh, lean cuts of meat over processed as they often have added sugars, and buy organic where possible. An approximate portion guide (uncooked weight) is 75–120g red meat, 100–150g poultry and game. Try to keep to a maximum of around three portions of red meat per week.

	Average portion	GL	Notes
Beef	75–120g	0	
Chicken	100–150g	0	A good choice – remove skin.
Kidney	75–120g	0	
Lamb	75–120g	0	
Liver	75–120g	0	
Pork	75–120g	0	

Sausages	75–120g	0	Stick to those with high meat content (90% plus) as they have less bread and fillers in them.
Turkey	100–150g	0	A good choice – remove skin.
Duck	100–150g	0	Good to add a bit of variety – remove skin.
Ostrich	100–150g	0	A nice change.
Game	100–150g	0	Occasional use – remove skin.

MEAT ALTERNATIVES

Soya and Quorn (vegetable micro-protein) are good low-GL choices. If you are following a vegetarian diet it's important to make sure you have a variety of protein sources including beans and pulses, nuts, dairy foods and eggs if you eat them. Try to have at least two different vegetarian sources of protein every day. An average portion would be 100–150g.

FISH

The omega-3 fats found in oily fish are great for taking care of you and your heart. They make the platelets in your blood less sticky and help prevent arteries from clogging. Approximate uncooked portion sizes are 150–200g white fish, 120–150g all oily fish, tuna and salmon, 120–150g shellfish. Aim to eat three portions of fish per week, with at least one being oily fish. Fish pâté is a great way of getting some of your oily fish quota and a healthier choice than some of the meat pâtés which can be very high in fat.

	Average portion	GL	Notes
Anchovies*	120–150g	0	
Caviar	1 tbsp	0	Bit pricey but low-GL!
Herrings*	120–150g	0	
Kippers*	120–150g	0	
Mackerel*	120–150g	0	
Pilchards*	120–150g	0	
Salmon* (canned or fresh)	120–150g	0	Very good for you.
Sardines*	120–150g	0	
Shellfish (prawns, lobster, crab, scallops)	120–150g	0	Good choices.
Tuna*	120–150g	0	A very healthy choice. However, only fresh tuna counts as oily due to the loss of oils during the canning process.
White fish	150–200g	0	A very healthy choice.

* denotes oily fish

VEGETABLES

Try to eat a rainbow of coloured vegetables every day to get a good variety of antioxidants, vitamins and minerals. Eat at least three portions a day if you can.

	Average portion	GL	Notes
Artichoke	80g	0	
Asparagus	80g	0	
Aubergine (eggplant)	80g	0	

Avocado	80g	0	A great 'power food' containing monounsaturated fat – a good source of vitamins A, C, E and potassium.
Beetroot	80g	4	
Broccoli	80g	0	
Brussels sprouts	80g	0	
Cabbage	80g	0	
Carrots	80g	2	
Cauliflower	80g	0	
Celeriac	80g	0	
Celery	80g	0	
Chicory	80g	0	
Collard greens	80g	0	
Courgettes (zucchini)	80g	0	
Cucumber	80g	0	
Endive	80g	0	
Kale	80g	0	
Kohlrabi	80g	0	
Leeks	80g	0	
Lettuce (all types)	80g	0	
Mange tout	80g	0	
Mushrooms	80g	0	
Okra	80g	0	
Onions	80g	0	
Olives	80g	0	A great, healthy snack.
Peas	80g	3	
Peas (marrowfat)	80g	4	
Peas (split yellow)	80g	3	

Peppers	80g	0	
Potatoes (baby new)	80g	6	Three or four new potatoes are fine.
Pumpkin	80g	3	
Radicchio	80g	0	
Radishes	80g	0	
Sauerkraut	80g	0	Contains cabbage and vinegar – available in jars from supermarkets. Vinegar lowers the GL of foods as it is acidic.
Spinach	80g	0	
Spring onions (scallions)	80g	0	
Squash (all)	80g	0	
Swede	80g	7	
Sweetcorn	80g	9	
Sweet potatoes	80g	9	Very nutritious and a good alternative to white potatoes.
Swiss chard	80g	0	
Tomatoes	80g	0	
Turnips	80g	0	
Watercress	80g	0	
Yams	80g	7	

Parsnips have a GL of 12 for 80g and so are classed as moderate – okay to use sparingly.

If you buy tinned vegetables check they have no sugar added – many do, surprisingly.

BEANS AND PULSES

Beans and pulses are fantastic sources of fibre – and have a low GL. The portion weight listed refers to the cooked weight. Don't be afraid to experiment – you don't have to stick with traditional recipes and food choices – go beanie mad instead!

	Average portion	GL	Notes
Baked beans	80g	4	You can buy reduced-sugar versions which will have a slighter lower GL.
Bean sprouts	80g	NT	Likely to have a lowish GL.
Black-eyed beans	80g	5	
Broad beans	80g	5	
Butter beans	80g	3	A great, low-GL, nutritious bean.
Chana dal	80g	2	A nutritious, very low-GL bean similar to chickpeas but sweeter. Available from Indian grocery stores and some supermarkets. Can be used in place of rice and pasta.
Chickpeas	80g	4	Becoming more popular now – healthy and low-GL.
Haricot (navy) beans	80g	6	
Kidney beans	80g	5	
Lentils	80g	3	
Lima beans	80g	5	
Mung beans	80g	5	
Pinto beans	80g	5	
Runner beans	80g	0	
Soya beans	80g	<1	A very low-GL choice.

FRUIT (Fresh)

The vast majority of fruits have a low GL. We have given the GL for a 120g portion but you don't need to weigh them – just guesstimate. You will see that not all the fruits have a GL rating. This is because they are so low in carbohydrates the GL is insignificant – berries are very low-GL and a brilliant choice. Stick to firm fruit – if it is soft and over-ripe, the GL will be higher.

	Average portion	GL	Notes
Apples	120g	6	
Apricots	120g	5	
Bananas	60g	7	(ripe)
(a small one)	60g	6	(yellow and green)
	60g	3	(green – under-ripe)

As you can see, ripe bananas have a much higher GL than under-ripe ones.

Blackberries	120g	0	
Blueberries	120g	0	
Cherries	120g	3	
Figs (fresh)	120g	NT	Likely to have a lowish GL.
Grapefruit	120g	3	
Grapes – green	120g	8	
Grapes – black	120g	10	
Kiwis	120g	6	
Lemons	0		
Limes	0		

Adding lemon or lime juice to recipes, salads and dressings helps lower the GL
  due to its acidity – so get squeezing!

Mandarins	120g	NT	Likely to have a similar GL to oranges.
Mangoes	120g	8	
Melons	120g	4	
Nectarines	120g	NT	Likely to have a lowish GL.
Oranges	120g	5	
Papaya (pawpaw)	120g	9–10	
Peaches	120g	5	
Pears	120g	4	
Pineapples	120g	7	
Plums	120g	5	
Prunes (pitted)	60g	10	
Raspberries	120g	0	
Rhubarb	120g	0	
Strawberries	120g	1	
Tangerines	120g	NT	Likely to have a GL similar to oranges.
Ugli fruit	120g	NT	Likely to be reasonably low-GL.
Watermelon	120g	4	

FRUIT (Dried)

To date, not all dried fruits have been tested but their GL values vary considerably. All dried berries such as strawberries, raspberries and blueberries are fine in small amounts. Pineapple and mango haven't been tested but should also be okay for limited use. Dried cranberries often seem to have sugar added, so be aware. Raisins have a high GL of 27 for 60g as do sultanas at 25 GL for 60g, so use very sparingly, if at all. Dried figs and dried dates also have a moderate-to-high GL score.

Tinned fruits are fine but make sure they are in their own juice rather than sugary syrups – check the label for added sugar.

	Average portion	GL	Notes
Dried apple	60g	10	
Dried apricot	60g	9	
Dried prunes	60g	6	

DAIRY AND ALTERNATIVES/OILS

Although butter has a bad reputation as it is a saturated fat, it is probably far less harmful than many of the low-fat spreads we have been encouraged to consume in its place for the last 20 years or so. Many of these low-fat spreads contained hydrogenated/trans fats, which health researchers are now linking to heart disease and cancer. As a result, governments throughout the world are now introducing either a complete ban on these fats, or drastically limiting the amount products are allowed to contain. Healthy alternatives to butter are the many olive oil-based spreads now available. Check the back of the pack to see if it contains trans fats/hydrogenated fats – some now advertise that they are virtually trans fat-free, which is a real health bonus.

	Average portion	GL	Notes
Butter	20g	0	Use in small amounts or preferably stick with the olive oil-based spreads – see page 203.

Cheese – all types	50–75g	0	Try and keep to no more than 50g of full-fat or 75g of low/half-fat cheese per day. Reduced-fat cheese is one of the few 'diet' products where the fat isn't replaced with sugar!
Cream	1 tbsp	NT	Squirty cream is a good choice – as it is aerated you will use less. It often contains a small amount of sugar but you can get sugar-free versions – check the label.
Crème fraîche	2 tbsp	NT	Good for cooking and sauces. Likely to be low-GL.
Eggs	1	0	Current nutritional research points to 1 egg per day being healthy, or an average of 6–7 eggs per week. Eggs are a very nutritious food. The long-standing concerns over the possibility that they raise cholesterol levels seem to have dissipated. Recent research carried out at Harvard Medical School recommends eating an egg per day.
Goat's milk	125ml	NT	A good alternative if cow's milk affects you adversely. Stick to ⅓ pint (175ml) per day. Likely to have a similar GL to cow's milk.
Ice cream	50g	3–8	A nice treat now and then – go for as natural as possible.

Mayonnaise	1 tbsp	0	Light or normal – a nice treat now and again.
Milk (cow's)	125ml	2	Stick to ⅓ pint (175ml) per day.
Olive oil	1 tbsp	0	A great healthy choice – use in salad dressings and recipes.
Olive oil-based spread	20g	0	A healthy choice with virtually no trans/hydrogenated fats.
Sheep's milk	125ml	NT	An alternative to cow's milk. Stick to ⅓ pint (175ml) per day. Likely to have a similar GL to cow's milk.
Sour cream	1 tbsp	NT	As a treat now and then – great with chicken fajitas, tomato salsa and guacamole. Likely to be low-GL.
Soya milk	125ml	2	An alternative to cow's milk. Look for sugar-free versions. Stick to ⅓ pint (175ml) per day.
Soya yoghurt	100g	6	These will vary depending on sugar content. Look for sugar-free versions.
Yoghurt	200g	2–4	These vary a lot in content – stick with sugar-free versions and as natural as possible. Or preferably add your own fresh fruit to natural yoghurt (such as bio and Greek).

NUTS AND SEEDS

Nuts are very nutritious but loaded with calories so stick to no more than a small handful of unsalted nuts a day. Many of the nuts listed on page 204 haven't been tested for their GL. However, as they are so low in carbohydrates they will have a low GL score. Recent research has shown that almonds actually lower cholesterol. You can use ground almonds instead of normal flour for baking.

	Average portion	GL	Notes
Cashew nuts	50g	3	
Flax seeds	50g	NT	
Hazelnuts	50g	NT	
Hemp seeds	50g	NT	
Linseeds	50g	NT	These can be ground and scattered over dishes as a healthy fibre boost, used in a seed mix (see recipe on page 121) or even sprouted! Whichever way you choose, always consume with plenty of water.
Macadamia nuts	50g	NT	
Pecans	50g	NT	
Peanuts	50g	1	Calorie dense, so go easy, and avoid the heavily salted or sugar-coated versions.
Pine nuts	50g	NT	Great toasted and used to top yoghurt or salads.
Pistachio nuts	50g	NT	
Pumpkin seeds	50g	NT	
Sunflower seeds	50g	NT	
Walnuts	50g	NT	

GRAINS

All weights are cooked weights unless otherwise stated.

	Average portion	GL	Notes
Buckwheat kasha	100g	10	
Bulgur wheat	100g	8	
Couscous	100g	7	A grain pellet normally made from durum wheat or buckwheat semolina.
Oat bran (raw)	10g	3	
Pearl barley	100g	5	A great low-GL choice to use instead of rice/pasta.
Popcorn (plain, microwaved)	20g	8	Avoid sweetened popcorn.
Quinoa	30g (dry weight)	9	Quinoa has a low GI of 51 but as it is high in carbs, the GL for 100g is a high 30. As it is a nutritious grain and a good alternative for those intolerant to wheat, we have included it – giving a smaller portion of 30g to bring the GL under 10.
Rice bran, extruded	30g	3	
Rye (whole)	30g (dry weight)	8	
Semolina	100g	4	Surprisingly low GL.
Wheat (whole)	30g (dry weight)	8	

30g of amaranth popped with milk has been tested as 21 – a high GL.

Spelt hasn't been tested yet so use sparingly for now.

BREAD AND CRACKERS

Although we give the approximate GL for 30g of bread/crackers below, a good guideline would be no more than one slice of bread per day for women (or two crackers) and two for men (or four crackers) while trying to lose weight. You won't find all these breads in your local supermarket, but they are now becoming more widely available. Try your local health-food shop. If in doubt go for the darkest, grainiest bread you can find. It will have more fibre, be less processed and have a lower GL than the highly refined white-flour breads. 'Wholemeal' bread has a similar GL to white as it is normally still highly processed. Gluten-free breads tend to have a higher GL as they are often based on corn flour. If you have a bread machine, there is a great, quick and easy, nutty seedy bread recipe on page 116.

	Average portion	GL	Notes
Dark Swiss rye	30g	9	
Oat bran and honey	30g	7	
Oatcakes	30g	8	
Pumpernickel	30g	5	
Rye crackers	30g	10	
Sourdough rye	30g	6	
Soya and linseed	30g	3	
Spelt multigrain	30g	7	
Sunflower and barley	30g	6	
Wholegrain	30g	7	
Wholemeal pitta	30g	10	
Wholemeal rye	30g	8	

PASTA AND NOODLES

Try and keep your pasta and noodles to smaller portions, as an accompaniment rather than the largest part of the meal. Make sure you cook them *al dente* (firm to the bite) as the longer they are boiled the higher the GL rises! Gluten-free corn-based pasta generally has a fairly high GL. Both our own experience and feedback from our fabulous GL dieters has told us that the amount of pasta and noodles you can eat and still lose weight varies significantly from one person to the next – so start with smaller amounts and see how it affects you. Mixing beans and pulses with pasta and noodles will enable you to have a bigger portion and lower the GL of the overall meal. All weights refer to cooked weights unless otherwise stated.

	Average portion	GL	Notes
Fettuccine, egg	100g	10	
Mung bean noodles, dried	100g	8	Available from some supermarkets, Chinese/Japanese grocery stores and health-food shops.
Ravioli	100g	8	
Rice noodles	100g	10	Quite widely available.
Soba noodles	100g	NT	These are also known as buckwheat noodles. Likely to have a lowish GL.
Spaghetti, white	100g	10	
Spaghetti, wholemeal	100g	9	
Tortellini, cheese	100g	6	

RICE

Rice is a high-GL food – if you choose to eat it, keep to a small portion of 75g (cooked weight). As with pasta, have it as an accompaniment rather than the main part of the meal. Mix it with beans and pulses or use pearl barley as an alternative as it has a GL of only 8 for 150g! Many of our low-GL dieters are getting very creative with pearl barley and using it in lots of recipes. See page 154 for our fabulous 'barleyotto' recipe.

	Average portion	GL	Notes
Brown rice	75g	9	
Wild rice	75g	8	

Long grain and basmati rice have a GL of over 10 even for 75g, so use the above two in preference.

SOUPS

Most soups are low-GL. Choose the most natural ones you can find. Fresh cartons are often the best choice – check tins as they sometimes contain hydrogenated/trans fats. Look for ones that include low-GL ingredients and skip the potato and pasta-based varieties. Or better still, make your own in the blender so you know exactly what's in them. Good soup choices would be tomato, tomato and basil/herb, asparagus, leek, broccoli, vegetable, lentil, pea, French onion – in fact, any low-GL vegetable as per the vegetable list on pages 195–7.

CHOCOLATE

Choose high-cocoa chocolate – 70% cocoa plus. This contains less sugar and, as it has quite a strong, rich taste, you tend to eat less. A few squares as a snack is a great healthy choice! There is a lot of recent research about the health benefits of the flavanols in cocoa too.

DRINKS

Choose juices that contain 100% fruit and no added sugar – preferably with bits of fruit or pulp still in it, which means more fibre and a lower GL. Limit your juice intake to 125 ml per day and mix with water to make a longer drink.

	Average portion	GL	Notes
Apple juice	125ml	6	
Carrot juice	125ml	5	A healthy drink.
Cranberry juice	125ml	8	
Grapefruit juice	125ml	6	
Orange juice	125ml	5	
Pineapple juice	125ml	8	
Pomegranate juice	125ml	NT	Not yet tested but likely to have a low GL – it is now becoming more widely available.
Tomato juice	125ml	2	A great choice.

The following drinks are fine and have a low GL. Drink as much water as you can but no more than one smoothie or yoghurt drink per day. Be aware that some of the coffee bar chains add syrups to their coffees which will make them high-GL – ask for plain coffee or a cappuccino.

	Average portion	GL	Notes
Diet drinks	1 can/bottle	NT	Normally artificially sweetened but still preferable to the sugar-filled versions.
Fruit tea	unlimited	NT	Likely to be very low-GL.
Herbal tea	unlimited	NT	Likely to be very low-GL.
Tea (black/green)	unlimited	NT	If you are drinking unsweetened teas without milk then you can have as much as you want.
Yoghurt drinks (sugar-free)	1 standard size	NT	

JAMS (JELLIES) AND SYRUPS

	Average portion	GL	Notes
Reduced-sugar jam	30g	5	
Maple syrup	25g	9	

SUGARS AND SWEETENERS

Artificial sweeteners such as aspartame, sucralose and saccharin are generally low-GL. Some people find them useful but we prefer to use fructose – also known as fruit sugar (not to be confused with high-fructose corn syrup) – as a more natural alternative to sugar. We don't recommend polyols such as maltitol as they can cause considerable gastrointestinal distress in some people – their GI/GL values vary considerably and they can cause immediate laxative effects! Some companies use polyols as sweeteners in their low-carb products and use the term 'net carbs', but this is controversial and confusing, especially as the effects of polyols vary from one person to the next. Unless specific products have been tested as low-GL, are made from healthy ingredients and shown to have little effect on your blood sugars, we wouldn't recommend them.

	Average portion	GL	Notes
Fructose	10g	2	Has a far lower GL than sugar, is sweeter so you can use a third less and good for baking (reduce cooking time as per pack instructions). Now available from most supermarkets. You can use in drinks as you would sugar but try not to sweeten drinks if you can – you will soon get used to less sweetness.
Honey	25g	10	Fine to use in small amounts.

SAUCES, DIPS AND DRESSINGS

When choosing ready-made sauces, dips and dressings, look for ones without added sugar, glucose/glucose syrup or dextrose. Better still, make your own with fresh ingredients so you know exactly what's in it! See pages 165–8 for inspiration.

Sauces – A sensible sauce portion would be 2–3 tablespoons per person. Most are likely to have a lowish GL, providing they don't contain added sugars (or only small amounts). The higher sugar is listed on the label, the more the product contains.

	Average portion	GL	Notes
Arrabiata		NT	
Asparagus		NT	
Balti		NT	
Black pepper		NT	
Bolognese		NT	
Chasseur		NT	
Cheese sauce		NT	
Forestière		NT	
Jalfrezi		NT	
Korma		NT	
Madeira		NT	
Madras		NT	
Mushroom		NT	
Napoletana		NT	
Pesto (basil, olive oil and pine nuts)		NT	There are lots of varieties in jars now – you can add a small amount of milk, cream or crème fraîche to make a sauce. No sugar added and likely to have a very low GL.
Puttanesca		NT	
Red pepper		NT	
Red wine and herbs		NT	
Roasted vegetable		NT	
Spinach and ricotta or nutmeg		NT	
Sweet pepper		NT	
Tarragon		NT	
Tikka masala		NT	
Tomato and basil		NT	

	Average portion	GL	Notes
Tomato and mascarpone		NT	
Watercress		NT	
White wine		NT	

You can easily whizz up a tin of tomatoes in the blender, add some herbs and
spices and a little crème fraîche to make a healthy sauce.
Some Indian sauces are quite high in fat, so go easy on those.

Dips – A reasonable portion would be a tablespoon. Here are some of our favourite shop-bought dips – check for added sugars as for sauces but many should be okay. The following are based on low-GL ingredients, so unless they are loaded with added sugar, they are likely to have a low GL.

	Average portion	GL	Notes
Cheese and chive		NT	
Cheese and onion		NT	
Garlic and herb		NT	
Guacamole		NT	Not tested but likely to be low as made from avocado, lemon juice, onion and chillies.
Houmous	100g	<1	Houmous, which is made from chickpeas, has a very low GL and is widely available – so enjoy!
Sour cream and chive		NT	Likely to have a low GL.
Tomato salsa		NT	Likely to have a low GL.
Tzatziki		NT	Not yet tested but no reason to avoid as it is generally made from low-GL ingredients – yoghurt, cucumber, garlic and olive oil.

Pâtés – Fish pâté is a great way of getting some of your oily fish quota and a healthier choice than some of the meat pâtés which can be very high in fat.

Dressings – A sensible portion would be a tablespoon. To add zing and make any salad scrumptious, you can't beat dressing it up! Again, making your own is ideal (see pages 165–8) but the range of shop-bought dressings is expanding rapidly – most have mainly low-GL ingredients but check the label for added sugars. Here are a few of our favourites.

	Average portion	GL	Notes
Avocado, mint and lime		NT	
Caesar		NT	
Chilli		NT	
French		NT	
Honey and mustard		NT	
Red pepper		NT	
Tomato and basil		NT	
Tomato and roasted onion		NT	
Vinaigrette		NT	
Yoghurt and mint		NT	

MISCELLANEOUS

	Average portion	GL	Notes
Coleslaw	1 tbsp	0	Can be high in fat but contains all low-GL ingredients – so a nice treat now and then.
Falafel	100g	NT	Made from chickpeas, broad beans, spices and coriander. You can buy falafel (round shapes) from most supermarkets now. Nice eaten hot or cold. Although not tested, it is likely to have a low GL.
Tabbouleh	50g	NT	Not tested but normally made from either bulgur wheat or couscous with lemon juice and herbs so should have a reasonably low GL.

HERBS AND SPICES

Use generously to add lots of flavour and interest to your food for both taste and decoration. If you can't be bothered to buy fresh herbs (you can freeze them), use dried instead. Garlic is great and so good for you.

" After I got married I started to enjoy the finer things in life: home-cooked food, entertaining and more holidays. Soon it all began to catch up with me. I'd never had to think about my weight before. In fact, I'd always been quite skinny. Before long my suits didn't fit and people at work kept telling me I'd got love handles! There was no way I was going to a slimming club but I just couldn't seem to shift the extra weight I'd gained on my own. Eventually my boss gave me his copy of *The GL Diet*. The fast-and-friendly plan suited me down to the ground at work, and my wife used the great recipes for our evening meals. I've lost 1st 4lb so far and am comfortably back into my suit trousers. "

John C from Bucks

Chapter 11

A GUIDE TO LOW-GL SHOPPING AND EATING OUT

NEVER shop when you're hungry!!

Are you a random shopper or a list-maker? We are a combination of both, and strongly suggest that before you start the first 7-day plan you become a list shopper and plan ahead. Once you've got the GL habit, you can be a bit more spontaneous. It would be really helpful to get rid of any naughty, high-GL foods before you start restocking with your low-GL goodies.

Our general bias is towards:

■ natural – the closer a food is to its original form the better
■ fresh – food retains more of its goodness the fresher it is
■ low hassle – we all have busy lives
■ low-GL – of course!

We do appreciate that we are all different and the time we want to spend preparing meals varies greatly. Not everyone has the desire to marinate for days or make their own spice blends ... apart from Deborah of course (she insists it's her meditation!).

First, we have included a basic shopping list for each seven-day plan for easy reference. If this looks like a lot of food to buy, bear in mind that you are also restocking your basic store cupboard. You may find you've already got many of the items on the list in your kitchen – so the shopping list is just to help you through the first week on whichever plan you choose. Of course, if you want to mix and match the seven-day plans you can create your own shopping list.

Seven-day Fast and Friendly Plan Shopping List

	Amount to buy	**Comments**
Almonds	1 small bag, unsalted	
Apricots, dried	1 small bag	A great snack.
Bacon	1 pack	Choose lean bacon.
Baked beans	1 small tin reduced-sugar (buy a few for the cupboard)	
Beef, minced. lean	200g	
Black pepper	1 shaker of roughly ground black pepper	Or buy whole black peppercorns and use grinder.

	Amount to buy	**Comments**
Bran sticks	Small bag/box	Sugar-free from health-food shops.
Bread, low-GL	1 loaf	See the food lists for guidance (page 206) – the seedier, nuttier and darker the better!
Cashew nuts	1 small bag, unsalted	
Cheese	1 medium pack of cheese slices	Buy your favourite full/half-fat hard cheese for the week.
Cheese, feta	100g (buy small pack)	
Cheese sticks	1 pack	Handy ready-wrapped cheese.
Chicken fillets	Packet of small fillets	Pre-cooked, spicy
Chocolate	1 x 100g bar for the week	Choose a bar with a cocoa content of at least 70%.
Coleslaw	1 large tub	
Cottage cheese	1 large tub	
Cream cheese	1 large tub	For snacks over the week.
Crème fraîche/cream	1 small carton	For recipes.
Egg mayonnaise	2 tbsp	Make your own or buy a ready-made tub.
Eggs	2 needed but buy 6	Hard-boiled eggs make good snacks.
Fettuccine	200g	Buy a packet of fresh pasta.
Fruit, apple	2	Snacks.
Fruit, cherries	1 small bag	
Fruit, grapes	1 small bunch	

	Amount to buy	Comments
Fruit, nectarine	1	
Fruit, peach	2	
Fruit, pear	1	
Fruit, strawberries	Small punnet	Use with yoghurt – any leftovers make a good snack.
Gammon steak	1 large per person	
Ham	5–6 slices from the deli	Choose good quality, lean ham.
Houmous	1 large tub	Use for snack and dips.
Lemon	1	Fresh or bottled juice.
Mayonnaise	1 small jar	
Milk (cow's, unsweetened soya, goat's or sheep's)	570ml–1.2 litres/ 1–2 pints	Up to 200ml/⅓ pint of milk per day, which is just over 1.2 litres/2 pints per week.
Oatcakes	1 pack	Look for sugar-free varieties.
Olive oil (extra virgin)	1 bottle	
Olive oil-based spread or butter	1 small tub	
Olives, black	100g for recipe but buy more	These are a great snack to keep stocked up.
Paprika	1 shaker of dried	
Parmesan cheese	1 tbsp dried or a piece	This comes up in quite a few recipes – buy a good-sized piece for the fridge as it keeps well or buy it ready-grated.

	Amount to buy	Comments
Passata	500g carton	Sieved tomatoes.
Peanut butter	1 small jar, sugar-free	Use sparingly as it's dense in calories.
Pesto	1 small jar	
Pine nuts	1 small bag	Use as required
Prawn salad in marie rose sauce	Buy 1 small tub (discard some of the sauce as there is usually a lot of it)	Or make up your own with prawns, mayo, 1 tsp tomato sauce and a squeeze of lemon juice.
Prawns	2 large handfuls (buy a small bag of frozen – take out and defrost as you need)	
Rye crispbread	1 packet (dark rye)	
Salad	2 cos lettuces or 2 bags mixed leaves	Use other lettuce if preferred but cos keeps better than bags of salad leaves.
Salmon fillets	2	Boneless, fresh or frozen.
Sauce (tomato-based)	1 jar pasta-style sauce	
Seeds, sunflower	1 small bag	A great snack.
Soup: asparagus; tomato and herb	1 carton of each fresh from chiller cabinet (or make your own up in the blender)	For lunch – choose your favourite soup from the food list – fresh cartons are the best option as tinned often contain hydrogenated fats.
Tomato ketchup		Use sparingly as has added sugar.

	Amount to buy	Comments
Tuna steaks	2	Use fresh or frozen.
Veg, avocados	2	Large, ripe (soft at each end when ripe).
Veg, cucumber	2 large for recipes and salads	
Veg, peas or petit pois	Buy 1 small bag of frozen and take out as needed	
Veg, red onion	Buy a few as they last for ages	
Veg, sweet potato	A few small ones	
Veg, tomatoes	• 1 beefsteak • 1 tub sun-dried • 12 vine-ripened tomatoes for recipes/ salads	
Vinegar, balsamic	1 bottle	
Vinegar, white wine	1 small bottle	
Yoghurt, natural	1 large tub	Natural bio or Greek in a large tub to decant or smaller individual serving tubs

Seven-day Veggie Friendly Plan Shopping List

Both the Veggie Friendly and Foodie Friendly plans use lots of fresh herbs and garlic. For convenience, you can use dried herbs or ready-made pastes. You may want to pick your four favourite fresh herbs – the recipes are pretty flexible and allow you to substitute one for another in almost all cases. Spices are also used – check your kitchen cupboards before you go as you might have quite a few of them already. We've included everything on these lists but you may want to customize them a bit to your taste and way of cooking.

	Amount to buy	Comments
Baked beans	1 small can	Reduced-sugar.
Beans, butter	2 cans	
Beans, haricot or kidney	1 can	
Bread, low-GL	1 loaf	The seedier, nuttier and darker the better!
Bulgur wheat	1 bag	
Cheese	• Individual pieces • Parmesan (can use ready grated) • 1 pack halloumi • 1 bufallo mozzarella • 1 pack feta	Buy your favourite full/half-fat hard cheese for the week, plus Parmesan to garnish some recipes.
Chickpeas	4 cans	
Chilli, green	1	Or use dried flakes/paste.
Chilli, red	2	Or use dried flakes/paste.

	Amount to buy	Comments
Crème fraîche/cream/	1 medium tub	For recipes throughout the week.
Eggs	6	Hardboiled eggs make good snacks.
Flour, 100% wholemeal/spelt/rye or buckwheat	1 small bag	
Fructose	1 box	
Fruit, apple	1	For snack.
Fruit, cooking apple	1	
Fruit, dried apricots	1 small bag	
Fruit, lemons	Large bag – slice fresh lemon into drinks too	Or use bottled juice.
Fruit, limes	2	Or use lemon.
Fruit, orange	1	
Fruit, pear	1	For snack.
Fruit, selection	For breakfast, day 3	Suggestion: berries and small banana.
Guacamole	1 tub	
Herbs, basil	2 bunches	Or use dried.
Herbs, bay leaf	A small jar	
Herbs, chives	1 bunch	Or use dried.
Herbs, coriander (cilantro)	1 bunch	Or use dried.
Herbs, dill	1 bunch	Or use dried.
Herbs, mint	3 bunches	Or use dried.
Herbs, parsley	2 bunches	Or use dried.
Herbs, rosemary	1 small bunch	Or use dried.
Herbs, thyme	1 small bunch	

	Amount to buy	**Comments**
Honey	1 small jar	
Horseradish	1 small jar	
Houmous	1 tub	
Lentils (green or red)	1 large bag	
Marmite	Pot	Or alternative savoury spread.
Muesli	1 pack/bag	No added sugar.
Mustard, grainy	1 jar	Pick your favourite.
Nuts, brazil	1 small bag	
Nuts, ground almonds	1 small bag	
Nuts, walnuts	1 small bag	
Oatcakes (sugar-free)	1 packet	
Oats, porridge	1 packet	Steel-cut have lowest GL.
Olive oil (extra virgin)	1 bottle	
Olive oil-based spread or butter	1 small tub	
Olives, black, fresh or tinned	1 large tub/tin	Good to keep a stock.
Pasta, wholewheat	1 small bag	
Peanut butter	1 jar	No added sugar
Pearl barley	1 packet/bag	
Pine nuts	1 small bag	
Rice, wild	1 small bag	
Salad, mixed leaves	2 bags	Or use your favourite lettuce/leaves.
Salad, rocket	2 bags	
Sausages, Quorn	1 pack	For breakfast, suggestion: 2–3 sausages per person.

	Amount to buy	Comments
Seeds, roasted	1 packet	There are a few roasted/ toasted seed mixes around, or quickly toast a few of your favourites.
Seeds, sunflower	1 small packet	
Sesame oil	1 small bottle	Use olive oil if preferred.
Spices, black pepper	Buy crushed black peppercorns or whole and use a grinder.	
Spices, cumin	Powdered or whole	
Spices, curry powder	1 packet/pot	
Spices, paprika	Powdered	
Stock, vegetable	Cubes or fresh	
Tabasco sauce	1 small bottle	
Tahini paste	1 small tube	
Veg, asparagus	500g	If not available use peas, sugar snaps or mange tout.
Veg, aubergine (eggplant)	1 medium	
Veg, avocados	5 large	
Veg, baby spinach	2 bags	Fresh or frozen.
Veg, bean sprouts	1 pack	Mixed sprouts, or sprout your own!
Veg, butternut squash (or other squash)	1	
Veg, cauliflower	1 medium	
Veg, celery	1 small bunch	

	Amount to buy	**Comments**
Veg, courgettes (zucchini)	500g	Fresh or frozen.
Veg, crudités	Carrot sticks, peppers, celery etc.	A great standby snack.
Veg, fennel	2 bulbs	
Veg, garlic	6–8 bulbs	You probably don't *need* this much, but it keeps well – you can use dried if you prefer.
Veg, greens	Selection for supper on day 7	Choose the greens you like best.
Veg, mushrooms	1 small pack	Choose your favourites.
Veg, onions/shallots	4 large onions or small bag of shallots	
Veg, onions, red	2	
Veg, onions, spring (scallions)	1 bunch	
Veg, peppers	4 red, 3 yellow/orange	Or use the ones in olive oil in jars and drain.
Veg, radishes	Small bunch	
Veg, selection	For day 2 dinner	Choose your favourite low-GL veg.
Veg, selection	For day 3	Choose your favourite veg for kebabs – see recipe on pages 88–9.
Veg, spinach	3 bags	Fresh or frozen.
Veg, sweet potato	1 small per person	
Veg, tomatoes, fresh:	20–24 medium 1 small tub/box cherry	

	Amount to buy	Comments
Veg, tomatoes, other:	1 small tub sun-dried 1 tube sun-dried tomato paste	
Veg, tomatoes, tinned	1 tin	
Vinegar, balsamic	1 bottle	
Vinegar, white wine	1 small bottle	
Wine, dry white	1 bottle	½ cup for recipe.
Worcester sauce	1 bottle	
Yoghurt, natural	2 large tubs	Natural bio or Greek – in a large tub to decant or smaller individual serving tubs.

Seven-day Foodie Friendly Shopping List

	Amount to buy	Comments
Artichoke hearts	1 jar or tin	Optional.
Bacon, lean smoky	1 pack	
Beans, butter	2 tins	
Beans, cannellini	1 tin	
Beans, haricot	1 tin	
Beef, lean, minced	600g	The meatball recipe works well with any minced meat.
Beef, lean, stewing steak	600g	This is for a casserole – will work with other meats too.
Bran sticks, sugar-free	1 bag	From health-food stores.

	Amount to buy	Comments
Bread	Make nutty seedy bread as per recipe on page 116.	Or buy the darkest, nuttiest, seediest bread you can find.
Bulgur wheat	1 packet/bag	
Capers, in brine	1 tin	
Cheese	1 packet	Buy your favourite full/half-fat hard cheese for the week.
Cheese, cream	1 small tub (need 150g)	
Cheese, feta	1 packet	
Cheese, goat's	1 pack	For snack.
Cheese, Parmesan	1 pack	This is used in a lot of recipes and keeps well in the fridge, or buy ready-grated.
Chickpeas	3 tins	
Chicken, large skinless breasts	4	
Chocolate (at least 70% cocoa content)	1 x 100g bar	For snacks.
Chorizo sausage	1 pack (need 125g)	Use lean bacon for a lower-fat/salt alternative.
Coconut, desiccated	1 packet/box	Unsweetened.
Coconut milk	1 tin	
Crème fraîche	1 tub (need 450g in total)	
Eggs	6	Hardboiled eggs make great snacks.

	Amount to buy	Comments
Flour, 100% wholemeal, stone-ground	1 bag	
Fructose	1 packet	
Fruit, apples	2	
Fruit, dried apricots	1 bag	
Fruit, grapes	Small bag	
Fruit, lemons	6–10, depending on how much you like them!	Or use juice.
Fruit, lime	2	
Fruit, melon	1 medium, or 1 bag frozen mixed	Any melon will work in the recipe, including watermelon.
Fruit, nectarines	1	There are 3 snacks in the 7 days that call for fruit – choose your favourites.
Fruit, papaya (pawpaw)	1	
Fruit, pear	2	1 for snack (or choose alternative fruit), 1 for recipe.
Fruit, summer berries	1 punnet/1 pack of frozen	
Herbs, basil	1 bunch	
Herbs, bay leaves	1 packet	
Herbs, chives	1 bunch	
Herbs, coriander (cilantro)	2 bunches	
Herbs, dill	1 bunch	
Herbs, mint	2 bunches	
Herbs, parsley	1 bunch	

	Amount to buy	Comments
Herbs, rosemary	1 bunch	
Herbs, thyme	1 small bunch	
Hoki, or any white fish (boneless)	2 fillets (1 per person)	This recipe works with any fish.
Honey, runny	1 jar	
Milk	570ml–1.2 litres/ 1–2 pints	Recommend up to 200ml/⅓ pint of milk per day, which is just over 1.2 litres/2 pints per week.
Mustard, grainy	1 jar	
Nuts: hazelnuts, almonds, brazil nuts, macadamias or walnuts (or a mixture)	1 bag	
Oat bran	1 packet	For the homemade bread.
Oatcakes	1 packet	No added sugar.
Oats, porridge	1 box	
Olive oil-based spread or butter	1 small tub	
Olive oil, extra virgin	1 bottle	
Olives	1 large tub or tin	Keep a good stock of these for snacks.
Peanut butter	1 jar	Unsweetened.
Pearl barley	1 packet/bag	
Pine nuts	1 bag	
Prawns, large peeled	15–20	
Salad	2 bags/leaves of your choice	Including lettuce, rocket, baby spinach, cos, romaine etc.

	Amount to buy	Comments
Salad, rocket	1 bag	
Salmon, smoked	1 small pack	This is for a breakfast with scrambled eggs – you can use lean bacon instead.
Seeds, linseeds	1 packet	Or flax seeds.
Seeds, pumpkin	1 packet	
Seeds, sesame	1 packet	
Seeds, sunflower	1 packet	
Smoked mackerel	1 packet	
Spices, allspice	1 packet	
Spices, black peppercorns	For grinding with a pepper mill	You can use mixed peppercorns in any of the recipes.
Spices, cardamom pods	1 packet	
Spices, chilli flakes or powder	1 packet	
Spices, cinnamon	1 packet	Powdered.
Spices, coriander seeds	1 packet	
Spices, cumin	1 pack	Ground or whole.
Spices, paprika	1 pack/jar	Or use smoked paprika.
Spices, peppercorns – mixed	1 packet	
Stock, vegetable or chicken	Fresh or dried	
Tabasco sauce	1 bottle	
Tahini	1 jar	For the homemade houmous recipe (page 142) – or buy ready-made.

	Amount to buy	**Comments**
Tuna steaks (fresh)	4	The recipe works well with other fish too.
Veg, avocados	2	
Veg, cabbage	1 small	Dark green if possible
Veg, carrots	2 large	
Veg, cauliflower	1 small	
Veg, celery	1 pack	
Veg, courgettes (zucchini)	2	
Veg, crudités	Selection	There are 2 snacks in the 7 days that include crudités – choose your favourite veg.
Veg, cucumber	1 large	
Veg, fennel	1 bulb	
Veg, garlic	10–12 bulbs	Depending on how much you like garlic! You can use dried if you prefer.
Veg, ginger	1 small 'hand'	Can use dried.
Veg, onion	1 bag (no fewer than 7)	Or shallots if you prefer.
Veg, onion, red	2	You can buy more as they keep well.
Veg, petit pois or peas	1 bag frozen (need 450g)	
Veg, red chilli	1	
Veg, red pepper	6 large	Or use the ones in jars in olive oil and drain.
Veg, spring onions (scallions)	Small bunch	

	Amount to buy	Comments
Veg, tomatoes	3 large	Or 1 small can of tomatoes.
Veg, tomatoes, sun-dried	1 large jar or tub	In olive oil.
Veg, tomatoes, tinned, chopped	2 tins	You can use passata in place of one of the tins.
Vinegar, balsamic	1 small bottle	
Vitamin C powder	1 pot	For bread-making.
Wine, dry white	1 bottle	For deglazing the pan.
Worcester sauce	1 bottle	
Yeast	1 packet	For bread (dried/fast active – specifically for bread machines).
Yoghurt, natural	3 large tubs	Natural bio or Greek – in a large tub to decant or smaller individual serving pots.

Once you are comfortable with the principles of low-GL, you can really expand your shopping list – there are so many more food choices.

Low-GL Convenience Foods

Although natural is always better, some processed foods can be incorporated into the GL diet. Healthy pre-packaged meals are on the increase as food manufacturers and

supermarkets start to react to their customers' prefer-
ences. We are not anti-ready-made anything so long as it
is healthy and nutritious, helps keep life simple and makes
lunchtimes and tired evenings more pleasurable. Here are
some guidelines for making sensible choices.

- Take a look at the list of ingredients. Generally
  speaking, the shorter the list, the more natural the
  product and the better it is. If the label reads too much
  like a science experiment, pop it back on the shelf and
  walk away! The nearer the top of the list an ingredient
  appears, the more of it there is in the product.
- Pre-packaged meals containing lean meats, poultry and
  fish are always the best savoury choices with low-GL
  vegetables and salads.
- Steer clear of convenience foods that include rice,
  pasta or potatoes or have sugar high up the list on the
  label. Sugar can also hide on the label as glucose,
  glucose syrup, high-fructose corn syrup (not to be
  confused with fructose), inverted corn syrup and
  dextrose.
- Processed meats such as ham, salami and sausages
  often have quite a high salt and fat content, so check
  the label. If you do indulge then be aware of what else
  you are eating that day – and drink plenty of water.
- Ironically, many products promoted as low-fat 'healthy
  options' tend to have added sugars to improve the
  taste.
- Some low-GL convenience sauces in jars are listed in
  the food lists, above. If you enjoy your Indian sauces

then keep the rice to a handful, and grab a tin of chickpeas for bulk instead. Drain and rinse them and throw in the microwave or a pan to heat through. You can combine them with a handful of rice, a delicious sauce and a crunchy salad and still remain low-GL.

- There is absolutely no shame in 'speedy veg' when you are short of time so buy those vegetable medleys and get microwaving, steaming or lightly boiling.
- Low-GL desserts are not so easy to find as the majority contain a lot of sugar. Fresh fruits, fruit salad and Greek yoghurt or crème fraîche are the best speedy options, or grab a piece of cheese with some grapes or your favourite fruits.

GL in a Jar

The deli counter and tinned food aisle can keep us in low-GL convenience for weeks! Here's a brief roundup of some low-GL jar and tinned heroes.

- Anchovies in olive oil
- Artichoke hearts in oil
- Capers in brine
- Chickpeas and all beans and pulses
- Chopped tomatoes, tomato purée & passata (sieved tomatoes)
- Flavoured oils and vinegars (see Chapter 9, pages 165–8)
- Guacamole

- Houmous
- Oils – olive, walnut, sesame, ginger, etc (see Chapter 12, pages 257–60)
- Olives of all types, shapes and sizes
- Pesto of all types
- Pickled cucumbers (there are some without sugar)
- Pickled hot or sweet peppers (again, without sugar)
- Pickled onions (without sugar)
- Porcini mushrooms, other dried mushrooms
- Peppers in olive oil
- Smoked mackerel in oil or tomato sauce
- Sun-dried tomatoes (in olive oil or dried)
- Tuna in olive oil, tomato sauce or brine
- Tzatziki

Herbs and Spices

Food tastes so good when it's herby or spicy! You don't have to spend hours sweating over a pestle and mortar creating your own blends as there are some brilliant ready-made spice blends available. You can buy ready-prepared garlic paste or crushed garlic in jars. Unfortunately, some herb pastes contain glucose or other undesirables so please check the label. Generally, you can use dried herbs as an alternative to fresh in any of the recipes. Or you can freeze leftover herbs for convenience (see Chapter 9). Another good trick is to buy olive oil or vinegar infused with the herbs, garlic or chilli your taste buds desire.

Where to Shop

Internet Shopping

Answer these two questions honestly:

1. How much do you really like grocery shopping?
2. And how good are you at resisting temptation?

If you're anything like us the answers are 'not a lot' and 'not great' – so what's the alternative – internet shopping!

Life as we knew it became easier when we found out that we lived in the right areas to get deliveries. It makes life *so* easy, and after the initial hassle of setting up your account you will have all the staple things you love in a 'favourites' list (how this works varies between supermarkets). It really is much easier to stick to what you actually need to buy and saves you from the temptations on offer when wandering around the supermarket or, worse still, when standing in the queue at the checkout! So give it a go – see you in the cyber-aisles!

There is a trade-off here – if shopping is one of the few times you get active or you find it a huge pleasure then please do not stop!

However, there are things you just can't get from the supermarket. We're great lovers of local health-food shops, farm shops, farmers' markets and high-street specialists – where practical and possible. It can be an eye-opening experience and great fun.

Health-food Stores

Local health-food stores and the increasingly popular organic food stores are usually veritable Aladdin's caves of the weird, wild and wonderful. Here you can find interesting flours (buckwheat, spelt, soya, gram, rye, nut), great grains, pasta alternatives, noodles, crackers, biscuits, sprouting seeds, soya products, tofu/Quorn, and good selection of nuts and seeds that are unsalted and generally not tampered with.

Farmers' Markets

Farmers' markets are wonderful resources for the wild, fresh and unusual – from venison and ostrich burgers to home-baked breads (you are likely to find some good seedy loaves amongst the baker's offering), cheeses fresh from the farm, and vegetables so fresh they are still in their mud jackets! Unfortunately, most of the natural jams and pickles will have as much sugar as the usual ones, so do read labels.

High-street Shops

The high-street butchers, bakers and fishmongers are dwindling. However, if you are lucky enough still to have them they can be a great resource. Local butchers can sometimes be coaxed into making a batch of high-meat-content sausages with little or no rusk, and talk you through the best lean cuts of meat available. They also often stock free-range eggs from local chickens. Fishmongers are another good resource to help you choose from their fresh sea harvest.

Eating Out, Low-GL Style

NEVER go out to eat on an empty stomach!

Here's a brief roundup of how to eat well and low-GL when you are out and about.

■ Have a good long drink of water before you go out – hunger can be confused with thirst. You could snack, too, before you go out – fruit, a piece of cheese, or something from the GL snack ideas in the food plans. You're much less likely to be tempted and overindulge if you're not faint with hunger by the time you arrive at the restaurant!

■ Enjoy going out – it's rare that the food is the focal point of going out. Mostly it's about friends, family, fun. Love the food and focus on the company.

■ Hardest of all will be the dinner party when there is no way of choosing the food you end up with on your plate. Eat the lower-GL part of the meal and a small amount of the high-GL stuff – so you can still be polite and feel virtuous.

■ Dessert is another tricky area, especially at a dinner party. Have a bit if you really feel you can't refuse, or wait for cheese, if that might be on offer. Best choices will be strawberries and cream, fruit salad, cheese with fruit or some plain ice cream.

■ In reality we are all going to be faced with situations where few low-GL options are available. Don't panic, enjoy the food and don't eat too much. Where possible, try and stick to the 80:20 guide (80 per cent low-GL, 20 per cent medium-high GL), and you won't go far wrong (see page 52).

■ Buffets are easy once you've got your head around the GL lists – choose salads, fish, meat, a few new potatoes, cheese, etc. Stay away from the pastry and sandwiches.

■ Booze makes weak-willed folk out of all of us so take it easy. You're delaying your weight loss when alcohol is involved, and are far more likely to say 'Oh go on then' as the breadbasket or dessert comes round. If you are drinking, match your alcoholic drink with a glass of water – you will end up drinking less alcohol and feel a whole lot better in the morning.

■ Waiters are so used to fussy eaters or special dietary needs these days that turning away the breadbasket or asking for salad instead of chips will not even raise an eyebrow.

■ Starters are often a good source of low-GL fare. So if the main courses are less promising have two starters

instead – the cupped hands rule applies wherever you
are (see page 191).

- Avoid bread, potatoes, pasta, rice, sugary and sweet
and sour sauces. Dive into salads (Caesar, chicken, ham,
egg, prawn, beef, avocado, Greek), veggies (soups,
crudités, extra veg instead of potatoes or rice), meats
(grilled, roasted, crispy duck, antipasto, carpaccio, chilli
con carne), fish (all fish), cheese, and fruit.

- Not all 'fast food' is bad these days. Thankfully many
fast food restaurants are actively adapting their
offerings towards healthier options. Beware of hidden
sugars and syrups in coffees, milk shakes, smoothies
and yoghurt drinks.

Chapter 12

LOVE YOUR FOOD *AND* YOUR BODY

Time and time again we have seen diets that forget about the complete nutritional package needed to achieve not only a healthy weight but also a healthy body. We believe passionately that any diet for life has to be sustainable, enjoyable, safe and nutritionally complete.

- We advocate a moderate intake of total fat, emphasizing the use of healthy mono and polyunsaturated fats as well as essential fatty acids.
- We are really keen that you watch out for the harmful effects of hidden hydrogenated fats.
- We are fruit and veg crazy! From day one we strongly recommend a minimum of five portions a day.
- We pull no punches about the excessive amounts of salt used in many processed foods, and recommend you include them wisely.
- And as with any effective long-term healthy-eating plan, we strongly recommend adequate fluid intake, particularly water, and increasing your activity level.

We've gone into a lot of detail about why we are so committed to the GL principles for weight loss. Let's spend a little time looking at the rest of the diet so you can be absolutely confident that your new way of life is healthy and nutritionally balanced.

We'll take different aspects of healthy eating in turn, but remember: a balanced diet can only be balanced when it is varied and mixed, so try not to get too hung up on individual foods.

We could write a whole book about healthy eating, so here is a brief summary of some of the main aspects we have taken into account when putting together your eating plans and recipes.

What's So Hot about Wholegrains?

A huge variety of cereal crops are grown for food throughout the world, including wheat, rye, barley, oats and rice. Grains are the seeds of cereal plants, and wholegrains consist of three elements:

- A fibre-rich outer layer (the bran)
- A nutrient-packed inner area (the germ)
- A central starchy part (the endosperm)

During processing or milling, the bran and the germ are often removed to give a 'whiter' refined cereal, which also happens to be a higher-GL cereal. Wholegrains, on the other hand, contain the whole grain, keeping all three layers together with their valuable concentration of nutrients and yes, you've guessed it, they tend to have a lower GL. Wholegrains are one of the foods we need as part of a healthy diet. However, most cereal foods eaten in the UK are refined, and our intake of wholegrains is very low.

Most of the goodness is concentrated in the outer bran layer and the germ of the seed so wholegrains contain up to 75 per cent more nutrients than their refined counterparts. Wholegrains are rich in fibre, both the insoluble type (which helps us keep a healthy bowel and avoid constipation) and the soluble type (which helps to lower cholesterol and promote healthy gut bacteria). Nutrients found in wholegrain foods include:

- B vitamins, folic acid and omega 3 fats
- Minerals such as magnesium, zinc, phosphorus and iron
- Antioxidants including vitamin E, selenium and copper, and phytonutrients such as phytoestrogens (lignans).

Evidence is mounting that eating wholegrains regularly as part of a healthy diet and lifestyle may help reduce the risk of many common diseases. It seems to be the complete package of nutrients working together which offers protection, rather than any one nutrient in isolation.

Recent research suggests:

- The risk of both heart disease and type II diabetes may be up to 30 per cent lower in people who regularly eat wholegrains. This benefit is not seen with refined cereals and is even greater than seen with fruit and vegetables.
- Some forms of cancer of the digestive tract may be lower with higher intakes of wholegrains. The fibre in wholegrains not only moves food along more quickly and easily, reducing the time that damaging substances are in contact with the gut wall, but also seems to provide a food source for friendly bacteria, enabling them to thrive and produce substances thought to be protective.
- Wholegrains help maintain a healthy body weight because they are often low-GL. As you already know, that means they make you feel fuller for longer, really helping keep those hunger pangs at bay.

In the recipes you will see that we tend to use mostly the lower-GL wholegrains. It's recommended that most of us should aim for two to three servings of wholegrains a day.

To increase your intake of wholegrains, try the
following:

- Swap white bread for wholegrain or rye/pumpernickel
  bread.
- Choose wholewheat pasta instead of white.
- Try eating tabbouleh, a popular dish made with bulgur
  wheat.
- Use pearl barley.
- Include oats in your diet.
- Substitute wholegrain flour for white flour.

When reading food labels, look for the word 'whole' in
front of the name of the grain, for example '100 per cent
whole wheat'. It's also a good idea to make sure that
wholegrain is listed towards the top of the ingredients list.
Even popcorn is classed as a wholegrain.

You will see from the low-GL food lists (Chapter 10)
that the wholegrain advice above fits in very well with your
new low-GL eating plan as wholegrains have a lower GL
than their highly processed counterparts!

Below is a list of some of the many wholegrain varieties
that can be used in a wide range of dishes – check out the
food lists for portion guidelines.

Amaranth

Amaranth was a staple of Aztec culture, known as 'king seed' and 'seed sent by God' as a tribute to its taste and sustenance. It is now becoming more popular and can be used in cereals, breads, muffins, crackers and pancakes.

Amaranth has a high level of complete protein. Its protein contains lysine, an amino acid missing or negligible in many grains. It is also gluten-free.

It has a high GL, even for 30g, so use sparingly or introduce small amounts when in maintenance mode.

Barley

Barley is one of the oldest cultivated grains. King Edward I standardized the inch as equal to 'three barley seeds'.

Hulled barley retains more of the wholegrain nutrients but takes ages to cook. Lightly pearled barley is more easily cooked. Pearl barley is a great low-GL choice and can be used in place of rice.

Buckwheat

Japan's soba noodles, Brittany's crêpes and Russia's kasha are all made with buckwheat. A cousin of rhubarb, buckwheat is not technically a grain at all. It's high in nutrients and has a nutty flavour.

Buckwheat is the only grain known to have high levels of an antioxidant called rutin – studies show that it helps improve circulation and prevent LDL (bad) cholesterol from blocking blood vessels. Buckwheat has a low GL.

Bulgur

When wheat kernels are boiled, dried, cracked then sorted by size, the result is bulgur. Bulgur is most often made from durum wheat, but in fact almost any wheat – hard or soft, red or white – can be made into bulgur.

Because bulgur has been precooked and dried, it needs to be boiled for only about 10 minutes to be ready to eat. This makes it an extremely nutritious fast food for side dishes or salads. Bulgur's best-known traditional use is in the salad known as tabbouleh.

Bulgur contains more fibre than quinoa, oats, millet, buckwheat or corn. Its quick cooking time and mild flavour make it ideal for those new to wholegrain cooking. Bulgur is a good lowish-GL choice.

Corn

Often dismissed as a nutrient-poor starch – a second-rate vegetable and a second-rate grain – corn is now being reassessed and viewed as a healthier food. Eating corn with beans creates a complementary mix of amino acids that raises the protein value.

A new study shows that corn has the highest level of antioxidants of any grain or vegetable – almost twice the antioxidant activity of apples! Corn on the cob and unsweetened popcorn both have a low GL – so enjoy!

Oats

Oats have a good flavour that makes them ideal for breakfast cereals. Unique among grains, oats almost never have their bran and germ removed in processing. So if you see oats or oat flour on the label, you're virtually guaranteed to be getting wholegrain!

If you like a chewier, nuttier texture, consider steel-cut oats, also known as Irish or Scottish oats. Steel-cut oats consist of the entire oat kernel, sliced into smaller pieces to help water penetrate and cook the grain. They create a great low-GL breakfast porridge.

Scientific studies have concluded that, like barley, oats contain a special kind of fibre called beta-glucan found to be effective in lowering cholesterol levels. Recent research indicates that oats also have a unique antioxidant that helps protect blood vessels from the damaging effects of LDL (bad) cholesterol.

Porridge is a great low-GL choice – and oats in general are great!

Quinoa

Quinoa (pronounced keen-wah) originates from the Andes, where it has long been cultivated by the Incas. Botanically a relative of Swiss chard and beets rather than a 'true' grain, quinoa cooks in about 10–12 minutes, creating a light, fluffy side dish. It can also be incorporated into soups, salads and baked goods. A small, light-coloured round grain, similar in appearance to sesame seeds, quinoa is also available in other colours, including red, purple and black. Most quinoa must be rinsed before cooking.

The abundant protein in quinoa is complete protein, which means it contains all the essential amino acids our bodies can't make on their own. Quinoa is gluten-free.

Quinoa is a very nutritious grain but has a highish GL. If you keep to 30g it brings the GL down to 9 – so enjoy in smaller quantities.

Rice

White rice is refined, with the germ and bran removed. Wholegrain rice is usually brown but can also be black, purple, red or any of a variety of exotic colours! Brown rice is lower in fibre than most other wholegrains. Rice is one of the most easily digested grains. It can be eaten by those who are gluten-intolerant.

Wild rice (see page 253) and brown rice have a lower GL than most other varieties, but use sparingly until you reach the maintenance stage.

Rye

Rye is a traditional part of cuisine in Northern Europe and Russia. It's unusual among grains for the high level of fibre in its endosperm, not just in its bran. Because of this, rye products generally have a lower GL than those made from wheat and most other grains.

The type of fibre in rye promotes a rapid feeling of fullness, making rye foods a good choice for dieters.

Spelt

One of the oldest cultivated grains, spelt is a distant cousin of modern wheat. With a distinctive, nutty flavour, spelt can be used in place of common wheat in most recipes.

Spelt is higher in protein than common wheat. There are anecdotal reports that some people sensitive to wheat can tolerate spelt, but no reliable medical studies exist currently to support them.

Spelt hasn't been tested for its GI or GL so use cautiously for now. It can be mixed with other flours for making bread.

Wheat

Wheat has come to dominate the grains we eat because it contains large amounts of gluten, a stretchy protein that enables bakers to create risen breads. Two main varieties of wheat are widely eaten: durum wheat is made into pasta, while bread wheat is used for most other wheat foods.

Bulgur makes excellent side dishes (see page 249). Wheat berries – wholewheat kernels – can also be cooked as a side dish or breakfast cereal, but must be boiled for about an hour, preferably after soaking overnight. Cracked wheat cooks faster, as the wheat berries have been split open, allowing water to penetrate more quickly.

A 30g serving of whole wheat has a low GL of 8.

Wild Rice

Wild rice is not technically rice at all, but the seed of an aquatic grass originally grown by indigenous tribes around the Great Lakes.

The strong flavour and high price of wild rice mean that it is most often consumed in a blend with other types of rice or grain. Wild rice has twice the protein and fibre of brown rice, but less iron and calcium. A 75g portion of wild rice has a low GL, as does brown rice.

Good Fats, Bad Fats

It's clear we all need to include some fat in our diets to remain healthy, but not all fats have the same effects on our health. Some are more beneficial than others and some are just downright unhealthy, especially when eaten in excess. The 7-day GL diet makes sure you get plenty of good monounsaturated and polyunsaturated fats and not too much saturated fat, but in this section we want to home in on two fats in particular – a real goody and a villain.

Fish Oils

We've all heard that eating fish, especially oily fish rich in omega 3 fatty acids, is good for us. Evidence first came from studies that looked at populations where fish formed a large part of the diet. The Inuit Eskimos and the Japanese, for example, eat more fish than we do in most Western countries, and for them heart disease is much less common.

Further research has shown clear benefits of eating oily fish:

- Lowers the risk of heart disease and blood vessel disease
- Helps maintain healthy joints
- Helps the healthy development of babies and toddlers

These benefits are thought to come from the omega 3 fatty acids, DHA and EPA. To get the maximum benefit we should try and eat oily fish regularly. These include:

- Fresh tuna
- Salmon

- Herring
- Mackerel
- Pilchards
- Rainbow trout
- Dogfish
- Prawns
- Crab

Although canned fish counts as well as fresh, some brands of canned tuna have the omega 3 oils removed during processing.

To get the most benefit, adults and children over 12 are advised to eat two portions of fish a week, one of which should be oily. This is equal to about 450mg EPA/DHA per day. Younger children will need less.

There has been a lot of publicity about chemicals that may be harmful in some kinds of fish. For most of us there is no risk from eating up to four portions weekly. However, if you are pregnant, breastfeeding or likely to become pregnant you should stick to a maximum of two portions weekly. Shark, swordfish and marlin may contain a concentrated source of mercury and so should be avoided by women who are pregnant or breastfeeding, and all children under 16.

There are currently no UK recommendations for supplement use, but the following guidelines may be useful, especially for vegetarians:

- Check labels for EPA/DHA content
- Stick to the amount found in 2–4 portions of fish (450–900mg EPA/DHA)

Trans Fats

Trans fats – or to give them their full name, trans fatty acids (TFAs) – are present in small amounts in a wide range of foods. They occur naturally in dairy foods and in beef, lamb and products made from these meats. Trans fats are also produced when vegetable oils are hydro-genated – a chemical process that hardens oils and turns them into solid or semi-solid fats. These hardened fats, usually referred to as hydrogenated fats, are widely used. For example, they can be used to make fat spreads, such as margarine, and are present in many baked products such as cakes and biscuits. They can also be produced when vegetable oils are heated for frying.

Trans fats, like saturated fats, raise blood cholesterol, particularly levels of 'bad' LDL cholesterol. They can also reduce levels of 'good' HDL cholesterol, as well as increase another form of blood fat called triglycerides. All these effects can increase your risk of heart disease. Gram for gram, the effects of trans fats appear to be worse than those of saturated fats, so they are potentially worse for our health.

Governments around the world are at last bringing in legislation to force food manufacturers to label products that contain trans fats and to limit the amount they can use, but currently you will still find many products containing these 'bad' fats on the shelves. This means you need to check labels for hydrogenated fats or hydro-genated vegetable oil. If a food contains either it will almost certainly contain trans fats too, and the higher up the list of ingredients, the more trans fat the food is likely to contain. In general, trans fats are found in cakes, biscuits, hard margarines, takeaways, pastry and pies, most of which you will be avoiding anyway.

Essential Oils

As well as fish oils, healthy fats can be found in natural oils from seeds, nuts and olives. These oils contain vitamins A, D, E and K plus monounsaturated fats, and some or all of the essential fatty acids (omega 3 and 6) and non-essential fatty acids (omega 9). They are anti-inflammatory, help protect us against heart disease, improve the condition of our nails, hair and skin, can ease depression, and may even help fight cancer.

Here are a few with a guide to making the most of them:

Almond Oil

Made from roasted almonds, almond oil retains the flavour of almonds. Use it in baked goods, pastas, drizzled over vegetables or on grilled bread.

Avocado Oil

Use extra virgin, cold-pressed avocado oil in salads. Best unheated, it contains vitamin E and omega 9 fatty acids.

Virgin Coconut Oil

Coconut oil has long been considered 'bad' – an undeserved reputation as it has tremendous benefits and many health claims attached to it. It also has a high smoke point, making it a good oil to use for frying. Coconut oil is also said to increase your levels of healthy lauric acid (which is known for being antiviral, antibacterial and antifungal), omega 3 and the GLA fatty acids. Be careful where you get it as some coconut oil is made from 'copra' – the husk – and is refined, bleached and deodorized. When it comes to coconut oil you do seem to get what you pay for.

Extra Virgin Olive Oil

Use for salad dressings and mix with balsamic or red wine vinegar. A good source of omega 6, extra virgin olive oil comes from the first pressing of the olives and is therefore the highest quality olive oil. This makes it more expensive so you could save it for dressings and use basic olive oil for cooking. The main difference is in the taste rather than the nutritional content.

Extra Virgin Sunflower Oil

A good source of omega 6, which can be used for salads or drizzled over cooked vegetables.

Groundnut Oil

Good for cooking as it has a neutral taste.

Hazelnut Oil

Like walnut oil, hazelnut oil tastes of nuts and is rich and flavoursome. A little goes a long way. Use in salad dressings with a bit of olive oil. It goes well with asparagus. You can also use it for baking.

Hempseed Oil

High in omega 3, 6 and 9, hempseed oil can be mixed with lemon juice for a salad dressing. Don't heat it.

Sesame Oil

Add a small amount to stir-fries at the end of cooking time, use in salad dressings or drizzle over steak. Don't heat it.

Walnut Oil

Walnut oil, made from roasted or unroasted walnuts, has a good rich flavour. In salad dressings, combine walnut oil with olive oil for a robust dressing. Walnut oil is especially tasty when paired with a good vinaigrette and used in a salad with toasted walnuts, fruit and cheese. Buy a small quantity as it doesn't keep well, and don't heat it.

Flax, Hemp, Evening Primrose and Pumpkin Oils

You can buy blends such as this now to add to salads and soups – high in omega 3, 6 and 9.

Rice Bran Oil

This can be used in salads and for cooking and frying as it has no aftertaste. Foods cooked in rice bran oil absorb less oil during cooking. It is a great source of vitamin E, antioxidants and micronutrients, has a very high smoke (burn) point, making it ideal for pan- or stir-frying, and has an excellent shelf life.

Flavoured/Infused Olive Oils

You can find some of these in supermarkets now or buy online. For example:

- **Chilli** olive oil – great with mozzarella cheese, tomato sauces or chocolate!
- **Garlic** olive oil – good for sauces, pasta, vegetables, fish or meat
- **Basil** olive oil – goes with rice and pasta salads, soups and tomato sauces
- **Rosemary** olive oil – good with potatoes, fish, beans, risotto or chocolate!
- **Lemon** olive oil – ideal for mayonnaise or with white or red meat or tomatoes

- **Ginger** olive oil – good for soups, fish, meat, rice and cakes
- **Porcini mushroom** olive oil – for risottos, sauces, soups and vegetables

Milk and Dairy

Milk and dairy products such as cheese, yoghurt, crème fraîche and fromage frais are great sources of protein and vitamins A, B12 and D. They're also an important source of calcium, which helps to keep our bones strong. The calcium in dairy foods is easy for the body to absorb.

Eating three portions of dairy products every day is a smart move to keep your bones in shape throughout life. An average adult should aim to eat 700mg of calcium each day.

Dairy foods are the richest source of calcium in the diet. One-third of a pint of milk, a small pot of yoghurt or a matchbox-size piece of cheese each count as one portion. There are other dietary sources of calcium such as broccoli, sardines, peanuts and cauliflower, but you need to eat large amounts of these foods to achieve the amount of calcium you get from three dairy portions. For people who cannot tolerate dairy foods, good choices are a calcium-enriched soya alternative, or goat's and sheep's milks.

Salt and Health

Eating too much salt can increase your risk of developing high blood pressure, which is directly linked to heart disease. It's a simple fact that lowering your salt intake reduces your risk, and it's easy to do. The average person's

---

Salty Sums

Salt is sodium chloride. As food labels often list both the salt and sodium content, it can be really confusing.

■ To convert salt to sodium divide by 2.5
■ To convert sodium to salt multiply by 2.5

For example:

■ 1g salt = 0.4g sodium
■ 0.8g sodium = 2g salt

Being realistic, most of us eat some processed food every day, but it is possible to choose lower-salt options without having to prepare everything you eat from scratch.

■ For ready-meals and sandwiches, choose foods with under 0.5g sodium (1.25g salt).
■ For individual foods like soups, sauces and snacks, choose foods with under 0.3g sodium (0.75g salt).

salt intake in the UK is about 9.5g or 2 tsp per day, and this needs to come down to 6g per day. Apart from adding salt during cooking and at the table, it's estimated that 75 per cent of our daily salt intake comes from processed food.

The main salty culprits are:

- Salty meats like ham, bacon, sausages and pâté
- Tinned, packet and instant soups
- Stock cubes, gravy browning and granules
- Smoked meat and fish
- Meat and yeast extracts
- Hard cheese
- Salted snacks like crisps, salted nuts and salted biscuits
- High-salt ready-meals, sauces and takeaways

Try and limit these salty foods to one serving per day.

What Else Can You Do?

- Use little or no salt in cooking.
- Try not to add salt at the table.
- Don't be fooled into using salt-replacement products – they usually just replace sodium with other salts like potassium, which have a similar effect on the body.

Water – Are You Getting Enough?

Water is essential for life. Each of us is made up of around 60 per cent water. The nutrients from our food are transported around the body by water, and most of the chemical reactions that go on in the body need water. All of these reactions produce waste products, and yes, you've guessed it, without water we couldn't get rid of any of that waste. Just like a car radiator, water flows through the body to help maintain the right temperature. We constantly lose water in our breath and through sweat, and if we don't replace the lost water we're in danger of overheating!

What Happens if You Don't Drink Enough?

A lot of people don't even realize they are dehydrated because they have become so used to feeling below their best. Dehydration can leave you feeling tired, constipated and nauseous, and can often result in frequent headaches.

How Do You Know if You're Dehydrated?

A good way of knowing if you are drinking enough is the colour of your urine! If it's pale and straw-coloured, you're okay. Any darker and you would probably benefit from drinking more.

How Much Do You Need?

In a moderate climate like ours, most of us need around six to eight cups or glasses of water each day to keep the balance right. In hotter climates this amount increases. Likewise, if we take part in strenuous exercise we need more water than usual to help us keep cool. A good guide is 1 litre of extra water for every hour of strenuous exercise.

What if You Don't Like Drinking Water?

Some people find water unpalatable but you can make it more interesting by adding slices of lemon and lime. Diluted fruit juice or a drop of no-added-sugar cordial is also a good way of jazzing water up if you find it boring. Fruit and herb teas make good hot drinks that will help you keep hydrated.

Do Tea and Coffee Count?

Drinks like tea and coffee and some fizzy drinks contain caffeine, which is a diuretic and can cause further fluid losses. However, drinking caffeinated drinks is better than not drinking at all. If you do drink lots of tea, coffee or cola, try swapping every other drink for water or squash with no added sugar. Start gently and build up your water intake every few days.

Do I Have to Drink Special Water?

If you prefer bottled or filtered water that's fine. But water straight from the tap is perfectly good too.

Vegetarian Diets

Being vegetarian means different things to different people. Some people include white meats such as chicken and fish (semi-vegetarian). Others avoid all meat but still enjoy dairy products and eggs (lacto-ovo vegetarian). Vegans avoid using any animal products from meat and eggs to leather shoes. Whichever type of vegetarian you are, you still need to make sure you are getting all the nutrients you need. An easy way to plan your diet, and the way we planned the seven-day plan for veggies, is to think about the food groups.

Fruit and Veg

Aim for a minimum of five portions of fruit and vegetables each day. Those containing vitamin C – including citrus fruits, berries, melon, tomatoes and pineapple – increase the absorption of iron from non-meat foods. Try and have a glass of orange juice with your breakfast, or include peppers and tomatoes with main meals.

Protein

Non-meat sources of protein are essential for vegetarians. They are also a source of iron and zinc. Choose from the foods listed below – eaten with wholegrains, the combined protein is similar in value to that found in meat.

- Soya-based foods, including tofu
- Beans, lentils and chickpeas
- Seeds, nuts and nut butters
- Eggs, if you eat them

Calcium-rich Foods

Don't forget dairy foods or their alternatives. Be sure to include these foods two to three times a day to keep your calcium intake up:

- Calcium-enriched unsweetened soya milk and orange juice
- Tofu
- Dried fruits, such as apricots
- Green leafy vegetables (not spinach)
- Nuts and seeds
- Tinned salmon and sardines if you eat fish

Vitamins

If you rarely or never eat animal foods you need to make sure you are getting enough vitamin D, vitamin B_2 and vitamin B_{12}. Vitamin D is generated by sunlight on your skin, but if you don't go outside much or have dark skin or cover your skin, you should include fortified spreads in your diet. For vitamin B_2 and B_{12}, try to have soya foods or yeast extract regularly, otherwise consider a B-complex supplement.

If you are vegan you should include small amounts of iodized salt or seaweed. It's also important to take extra care during pregnancy, breastfeeding, weaning or in childhood to make sure all nutritional needs are being met. You may need to seek additional dietary advice at these times from your dietician, doctor or health visitor.

Making Sense of Food Labels

The label on most foods and drinks can provide useful information about their nutritional content. Amounts are given per 100g of food and may also be provided per serving of the product, so you can work out how much energy, protein, fat and sugar you will be getting. Some labels give further information, such as types of fat, dietary fibre and sodium.

Energy: It can be expressed as kJ (kilojoules) or as kcals (kilocalories). Strictly speaking a kilocalorie is equivalent to 1000 calories, but in everyday language, the term calorie tends to be used for both measures.

Protein: It is very rare in the UK for anyone not to be eating enough protein, the best rule for health is to make sure you get your protein from as many different sources as possible.

Carbohydrate: It includes both sugars and starches. The figure given for sugars includes both added sugar and natural sugar (i.e. fruit sugar).

Fat: There are three types of fat listed on food labels: saturates, polyunsaturates and monounsaturates. The label will show the total amount of fat, and may provide information on the different types as well. Hydrogenated/trans fats are rarely listed here, you need to check the ingredients list.

Fibre: We should be aiming to eat about 18g of fibre every day, and this should be a mix of insoluble fibre from wholegrains, for gut health, and soluble fibre from oats, beans and fruits and vegetables, to help control high levels of cholesterol.

Nutritional information	per portion	per 100g
Energy	1462kJ	975kJ
	351kcal	234kcal
Protein	9.0g	6.0g
Carbohydrate	28.2g	18.8g
of which sugars	3.0g	2.0g
of which starch	25.2g	16.8g
Fat	22.3g	14.0g
of which saturate	7.6g	5.1g
of which monounsaturates	10.9g	7.3g
of which polyunsaturates	2.7g	1.8g
Fibre	1.6g	1.1g
Sodium	0.6g	0.4g
Per portion	351kcals	22.3g fat

Salt/sodium/sodium chloride: Food labels often list both the salt and sodium content – it can be really confusing.
To convert salt to sodium, divide by 2.5
To convert sodium to salt, multiply by 2.5
For example:
1g salt = 0.4g sodium
0.8g sodium = 2g salt
You are aiming to keep your salt intake to 6g per day.

What about Health Claims?

There are many low-fat products on the market. Some, such as low-fat cheese and yoghurt, are fine. Others, however, may have replaced the fat with extra sugar, and so will probably be high-GL. Exercise caution here and check your labels.

Here is an explanation of what commonly-used nutrition claims actually mean:

- **Low fat:** indicates the food contains less than 3g fat per 100g/100ml of the food.
- **Reduced fat:** the food must contain 25 per cent less than a similar standard product. It doesn't mean it is low fat.

- **Less than 5% fat or (95% fat-free):** indicates the food contains less than 5g fat per 100g. For example, if you bought a ready-meal which had this claim and the serving was 400g, then the whole meal would contain 20g fat.
- **X% less fat than the standard product:** shows the fat reduction made to a product compared to a standard named product, such as 20 per cent less fat than a comparable product.
- **No added sugar:** no sugars from any source have been added. May still contain a lot of natural sugar, however.
- **Low sugar:** contains no more than 5g of sugar per 100g/100ml of food.
- **Reduced sugar:** must contain 25 per cent less sugar than the regular product. Be aware that, despite this, the product may still be high in sugar.

As you can see, labelling can be very confusing. Different types of fats and sugars are often listed under different names. It is important to know the GL of a product so that we understand how it will affect us after we have consumed it.

❝ This new way of eating has worked brilliantly for me and I haven't felt the need to revert to my old eating habits. I've discovered lots of different types of food and rarely feel hungry – which is new for me. My partner and I started this new way of eating at the same time and we have both lost weight. We still eat out but stick to the guidelines – that way we don't feel we are missing out on the dining experience.

I have lost just under one-and-a-half stones in only one month and I feel so much better in myself. My skin looks great, I feel fitter and everyone keeps telling me how young I look! ❞

Jean A from East London

PART V

FURTHER INFORMATION

This section takes things a step further by providing you with some additional information on GL.

You'll find:

- A review of international research
- Answers to many of your questions

" I found the GL book by accident while looking for the GI one my GP had recommended. As a busy cardiac nurse, I was disgusted to find myself very overweight with high blood pressure, raised cholesterol and hypoglycaemia.

After reading the book from cover to cover I initially decided to give it a go for a couple of weeks. That was 10 weeks ago and I haven't looked back since. I'm now 11lb lighter – a very healthy weight loss – and this is the first time in my life that I don't feel I'm on a diet! I haven't had a hypoglycaemic attack since starting the plan; my cholesterol is falling and so is my blood pressure. All in all I am much healthier and happier. This is definitely a life-changing plan. "

Melanie G from Torquay, Devon

Chapter 13

THE EVIDENCE – RESEARCH THAT SHOWS LOW-GLYCAEMIC DIETS WORK

Comparison of High- and Low-glycaemic Diets over Two 12-week Periods

'The low-glycaemic diet testers lost 2kg more weight in the first 12-week period and 3kg more in the second 12-week period than the high-glycaemic dieters.'

Source: Slabber et al., *American Journal of Clinical Nutrition*, 1994

'A study of 42,759 male health professionals … showed that a high-GL diet increased the risk for men to get type II diabetes.'

Source: *Diabetes Care*, April 1997

Twelve pregnant women ate either a high-glycaemic or low-glycaemic diet during pregnancy.

'The women on the low-glycaemic diet gained 12kg compared with the women on the high-glycaemic diet who gained 20kg.'

Source: Clapp J, *Archives of Gynaecology and Obstetrics*, 1997

'Research into dietary fibre, Glycaemic Load and diabetes risk in women revealed that the dietary Glycaemic Index, as well as the dietary Glycaemic Load, was positively associated with risk of diabetes. The more high-glycaemic carbohydrates consumed, the greater the incidence of diabetes. Fibre intake was associated with a decreased risk of diabetes. Researchers concluded that diets with high-glycaemic load and low fibre intake increase risk of diabetes in women. Further, they suggest that by consuming minimal amounts of refined carbohydrates, the incidence of diabetes can be reduced.'

Source: *Journal of the American Medical Association*, 277(6), 1997

Over a four-month period, 109 overweight children ate either a low-glycaemic or a low-fat diet.

'Of the children on the low-glycaemic diet, 17 per cent reduced their BMI (body mass index) by three units, compared to only 2 per cent in the low-fat group.'

Source: Spieth et al., *Archives of Pediatric and Adolescent Medicine*, 2000

A diet trial in 31 clinics across Europe looked at 1,500 adults with type I diabetes.

'The GI of the diet correlated positively with waist circumference in men.'

This means the lower the GI of the diet, the lower the waist circumference. This is significant because the higher the waist circumference, the higher the risk of cardiovascular disease.

Source: Buyken et al, *International Journal of Obesity*, 2001

'When dietary Glycaemic Load was assessed by a food frequency questionnaire in postmenopausal women, the results revealed that as Glycaemic Index, carbohydrate intake and Glycaemic Load increased, levels of HDL ("good") cholesterol decreased and triglycerides increased. The relationship between Glycaemic Load and elevated triglycerides was greater in women who were overweight. Researchers concluded that this study supports the physiologic relevance of the Glycaemic Load as a potential risk factor for coronary artery disease in women, particularly those prone to insulin resistance.'

Source: *American Journal of Clinical Nutrition*, 73(3), 2001

'Researchers have found that people who eat "low-quality carbohydrates" have high levels of C-reactive protein (CRP), a powerful promoter of inflammation. Growing research indicates that inflammation of blood vessels is at the root of heart disease and many other common degenerative diseases. High CRP levels increase the risk of heart attack 4.5 times. Women who consumed large amounts of potatoes (mostly mashed and baked), breakfast cereals, white bread, muffins and white rice had the highest CRP levels. It is conceivable that high-glycaemic foods may also stimulate the inflammation characteristics of arthritis, asthma and many other diseases.'

Source: *American Journal of Clinical Nutrition*, 2002, 75:492–498

Glycaemic Load Comes of Age

'Calculated GL can predict the glycaemic response to individual foods across a wide range of portion sizes and calls into question the conventional strategy of "carbohydrate counting" for controlling blood glucose levels. GL would seem to be a much better predictor than carbohydrate amount alone, because similar glycaemic responses were observed among foods differing in available carbohydrate by more than twofold.'

Source: David S Ludwig, *J Nutr*. Sept 2003, 133 (9): 2695–2696

'We speculate that the prolonged satiety associated with low-GI foods may prove an effective method for reducing caloric intake and achieving long-term weight control.'

Source: *Pediatrics*, 111(3), 2003

'Sixteen testers followed either a low-GL diet or a low-fat diet for 12 months.

'The low-GL diet testers lost more body fat and kept it off, whereas the low-fat testers gained body fat during the second six-month period.'

Source: Byrnes et al., *British Journal of Nutrition*, 2003

'Seventeen overweight men ate one of four different diets for a period of 24 days.

'Despite efforts to maintain identical energy intakes, men on the low-glycaemic diet lost weight compared to those on the high-glycaemic, high-fat and high-sugar diets.'

Source: Byrnes et al., *British Journal of Nutrition*, 2003

'Pregnant women who eat sugary or highly processed foods, known as high-GI foods, may have an increased risk of neural tube defects such as spina bifida in their newborns. The risk doubled for women who ate a lot of these foods, and amongst obese women the risk quadrupled.'

Source: *American Journal of Clinical Nutrition*, November 2003

'Two groups of rats were fed diets made up of 69 per cent carbohydrates. One group was fed high-GI carbohydrates and the other group low-GI carbohydrates. After 18 weeks the high-GI group had 71 per cent more body fat and 8 per cent less lean body mass than the low-GI group. The high-GI group also had higher levels of triglyceride blood fats, another heart disease risk factor in humans.

'In a further study, two groups of mice were put on either a low- or high-GI diet. After nine weeks, the high-GI group had 93 per cent more body fat than the mice on the low-GI diet.'

Source: 'Effects of dietary Glycaemic Index on adiposity, glucose homoestasis and plasma lipids in animals', *Lancet*, 2004

'In type II diabetics, a low-glycaemic diet significantly lowers fasting serum fructosamine and cholesterol levels after only two weeks.'

Source: TM Wolever, DJ Jenkins et al., Dept of Nutritional Sciences, Faculty of Medicine, University of Toronto, Canada

'Dietary Glycaemic Load has been significantly associated with an increased risk of colorectal cancer. Researchers speculate that a diet prominent in foods with high glycaemic indices, like white bread and white rice, affect insulin factors or exacerbate inflammatory responses and, thereby, increase the cancer risk.'

Source: Women's Health Study in *Journal of the National Cancer Institute*, February 2004

'A study of children found that those eating a low-GI breakfast tended to eat more moderately throughout the day, while those eating a high-GI breakfast were more likely to be hungry by lunchtime.'

Source: *Pediatrics*, Nov. 2004, (112 (5):e414)

'"The simple change from white bread to lower-GI bread within a high carbohydrate diet could reduce the risk of diabetes," according to Australian researchers. For many people, just swapping "bread type may be a more accept-able dietary change than one requiring a whole new eating pattern". The researchers, who included Allison Hodge of the Cancer Council in Victoria, followed the diets and health records of more than 36,000 men and women in Australia for four years. They found white bread was the food most strongly related to diabetes incidence – partici-pants who ate the most white bread (more than 17 slices per week) had the highest risk of diabetes.'

Source: *Diabetes Care*, November 2004

Low-GL Diet Can Help Dieters Get Past Plateau

'After they lose some weight, people often hit a point where it becomes harder to lose more weight. This is because as people lose weight, they actually burn fewer calories. So, the more weight a person loses, the fewer calories they burn. Researchers wanted to find out if a diet low in carbohydrates that are easy to digest (a low-GL diet) is better at helping dieters keep losing weight than a low-fat diet. Low-GL foods include prunes, barley, beans apples and other foods.

'Researchers studied 39 overweight or obese adults aged 18 to 40. Each person had to lose 10 per cent of his or her body weight at the beginning of the study to stay in the study. People in the study were put into two groups and given two different calorie-restricted diets: one low-fat and the other low-GL.

'The study found that people on the low-GL diet burned more calories, even at rest, than people on the low-fat diet. Also, people in the low-GL group reported less hunger than those in the low-fat group.

'Although people in both groups lost about the same amount of weight, the low-GL diet had other benefits: less heart disease risk, lower insulin resistance, lower lipids and fewer signs of inflammation. A low-GL diet (or a diet low in carbohydrates that are easy to digest) may help overweight people keep losing weight better than a low-fat diet.

'Dieters who have trouble keeping weight off, or who can't seem to lose beyond a certain point, may want to try a low-GL diet.'

Source: 'Effects of a low glycaemic load diet on resting energy expenditure and heart disease risk factors during weight loss', *Journal of the American Medical Association*, 292:2482–2490, 2004 (as reported by American Diabetes Association)

Low-GL Diet May Improve Ability to Stay on Diet Longer

'Low-GL diets, those low in sugars with moderate levels of carbohydrates and not as low in fat and protein, may lower metabolism less when compared with low-fat diets, making the dieters feel less tired, cold and hungry, as well as improve cardiovascular risk factors.

'Reduction in GL may aid in the prevention or treatment of obesity, cardiovascular disease and type II diabetes. For example, insulin resistance decreased by more than twice as much with weight loss in the low-GL versus the low-fat group.

Source: *Journal of the American Medical Association*, November 2004

'"Composition of diet may impact how dieters respond to weight loss," said lead researcher, Mark Pereira, Ph.D., assistant professor in epidemiology at the University of Minnesota. "On a typical low-fat diet, the participants tended to experience more perceived hunger and a slower metabolic rate, which may make it more difficult to stay on the diet, while those on the low-GL diet did not feel as hungry and had a faster metabolic rate."

'"In addition, the low-GL diet had beneficial effects on several obesity-related risk factors compared with a low-fat diet that was consistent with current nutritional guidelines."'

Source: medicalnewstoday.com, 24 November 2004

Low-glycaemic Diet May Help Keep Weight off and Raise Metabolism

'Dieters have higher metabolism and feel less hungry. Preliminary data from Children's Hospital Boston and Brigham and Women's Hospital suggest that weight-loss diets may be more effective when dieters seek to reduce GL – the amount their blood glucose rises after a meal – rather than limit fat intake. The findings indicate that a low-GL diet may overcome the body's natural tendency to slow metabolism and turn on hunger cues to "make up" the missing calories.

'The low-GL diet reduces carbohydrates that are rapidly digested and raise blood sugar and insulin to high levels – such as white bread, refined breakfast cereals and concentrated sugars. Instead, it emphasizes carbohydrates that release sugar more slowly, including wholegrains, most fruits, vegetables, nuts and legumes. "Our data suggest that the type of calories consumed – independent of the amount – can alter metabolic rate," says Dr David Ludwig, director of the Optimal Weight for Life (OWL) obesity program at Children's Hospital Boston and the study's senior investigator. "That hasn't been shown before. The idea that 'a calorie is a calorie is a calorie' doesn't really explain why conventional weight-loss diets usually don't work for more than a few months."

'Ludwig and colleagues randomized 46 overweight or obese adults aged 18 to 40 to consume one of two diets: a standard low-fat diet or a low-GL diet. Both diets provided approximately 1500 calories/day and were designed to produce a 10 per cent weight loss in 6 to 10 weeks. However, the low-GL diet was higher in fat and made various carbohydrate substitutions, such as steel-cut oats instead of instant oatmeal, blueberries instead of raisins, and cracked-wheat bread instead of tortilla chips.

'The 39 subjects who remained in the study succeeded in losing about 10 per cent of their initial body weight. The low-GL dieters had smaller decreases in resting energy expenditure (averaging 96 kcal/day, or 5.9 per cent) than the low-fat dieters (averaging 176 kcal/day, or 10.6 per cent), meaning their metabolism did not slow as much. They also reported less hunger each day while on their diets.

'"Almost anyone can lose weight in the short term – very few keep it off in the long term," says Ludwig. "That's given rise to the notion that the body has a 'setpoint' – and that when you diet, internal mechanisms work to restore your weight to that setpoint. A low-GL diet may work better with these internal biological responses to create the greatest likelihood of long-term weight loss."

'Confirming other research, Ludwig's team also found that the low-GL group had significantly greater improvements in insulin resistance (a risk factor for diabetes) and serum triglyceride and C-reactive protein levels (risk factors for cardiovascular disease).'

Source: medicalnewstoday.com,
24 November 2004

'Studies from the Harvard Medical School of Public Health indicate that the risks of diseases such as type II diabetes and coronary heart disease are strongly related to the GI of the overall diet. In 1999, the World Health Organization (WHO) and Food and Agriculture Organization (FAO) recommended that people in industrialized countries base their diets on low-GI foods in order to prevent the most common diseases of affluence, such as coronary heart disease, diabetes and obesity.'

**Source: Professor Jennie Brand-Miller,
University of Sydney, 2004**

'Replacing refined carbohydrates with high-fibre, low-GI carbs may help reduce the risk of haemorrhagic stroke in women, according to researchers including Dr Walter Willett from Harvard University and Brigham and Women's Hospital. Haemorrhagic stroke (also known as cerebral haemorrhage) occurs when a blood vessel in the brain breaks or ruptures. A high intake of refined carbohydrate may increase the risk of haemorrhagic stroke in women, particularly women who are overweight or obese. These results "may have implications for preventing stroke in Asian countries with a higher rate of haemorrhagic stroke and a higher intake of carbohydrate," say the authors.'

Source: *American Journal of Epidemiology*, 2005

'Researchers at the University of Massachusetts Medical School (UMMS) analysed the eating habits of 572 people in Massachusetts and found a clear link between the intake of certain carbohydrate foods and higher body mass index

(BMI). They found that people who ate more refined grains, starchy vegetables, white flour and similar carbohydrates were significantly heavier than people who ate foods with "good carbohydrates" such as wholegrains, non-starchy vegetables, nuts and seeds. It wasn't the total amount of carbohydrates that made the difference; it was the type of carbohydrates eaten that tipped the scales. "There are many factors involved in obesity, but our study found a clear association with eating certain carbohydrates and body weight," said Yunsheng Ma, MD, PhD, assistant professor of medicine at UMMS.'

> Source: *American Journal of Epidemiology*,
> February 2005

'The scientific benefits of eating low-GI foods as part of a balanced diet are becoming increasingly clear, according to Dr Gary Frost, head of the Department of Nutrition and Dietetics at Hammersmith Hospitals NHS Trust. Hammersmith researchers found that eating just one extra low-GI item per meal can reduce the risk of metabolic syndrome. They measured the blood glucose levels of nine people on normal diets, and then put them on a low-GI diet involving replacing one low-GI item per meal for two weeks. When the readings were taken again, eight out of nine had lower blood glucose readings. According to Dr Frost, "Any diet measure that was going to be successful needed to be realistic and manageable. The low-GI diet (has) the potential to have a huge impact because of its simplicity."'

> Source: *British Journal of Nutrition*
> (2005) 93, 179–182

'"A diet focused on glycaemic index may be easier to follow than diets restricted in either fat or carbs," reports David S. Ludwig, MD, PhD, associate professor of paediatrics at Children's Hospital, Boston. "And there seems to be an additional benefit in reducing the risk of chronic disease." In a 12-month study he found that 11 obese 30-year-olds on a "slow-carb" diet lost similar amounts of weight to 12 of their obese peers on a conventional low-fat diet. But they also lowered their risk of heart disease. They didn't avoid fats or carbs. They didn't count calories or eat prepackaged foods. The key was eating plenty of satisfying foods that the body can't quickly convert into sugar – what are called slow- or low-GI carbs.'

Source: *American Journal of Clinical Nutrition*,
May 2005

'An ad libitum low-GL diet may be more efficacious than a conventional energy-restricted, low-fat diet in reducing cardiovascular disease risk.'

Source: *American Journal of Clinical Nutrition*,
May 2005

Chapter 14

YOUR QUESTIONS ANSWERED

Why haven't all foods been tested for their GI and GL?

Testing has to be done in a controlled laboratory setting. It involves taking blood samples from a group of volunteers and comparing their blood glucose levels after eating the test food, and again after eating the same amount of available carbohydrates from glucose. Testing is therefore both expensive and time consuming to carry out. To begin with, scientists just tested basic carbohydrate foods but now many food manufacturers are starting to have their own products tested and to show their glycaemic response on packaging. We think this is a good move and will help give us more information about the food we eat and how our bodies react to it. More foods are being tested all the time – we regularly update information on our website www.dietfreedom.co.uk

Why don't I need to count calories on the low-GL diet?

By reducing the 'overall' GL of our daily diets we can help prevent fat storage. Providing we stick to the few quantity recommendations provided on certain foods and eat until we are satisfied rather than 'stuffed' there is no need to count calories. Anyway it's so boring – life and food are to enjoy after all! You obviously can't eat loads of calorie-dense foods like nuts and cream every day and expect to lose weight, but we now know that calories are only part of the equation, and simply reducing them is not the weight-loss Holy Grail it promised to be.

Do I have to count GL points?

No, definitely not. Many of our Diet Freedom Fighters are former points and calorie counters. Although it takes a while to kick the habit, the diet freedom that ensues is just brilliant to behold. Lowering the overall GL of your diet by using the 7-day plans and the food lists will get you on the road to eating healthily and losing weight at the same time – a double whammy. That really is all you need, along with a bit of a boost to your activity level, like our walking challenge in Chapter 2. Eating a low-GL diet will help to regulate your appetite naturally and prevent those blood sugar lows after eating high-GL foods that have you heading for the biscuit tin or rooting through the cupboards for something sugary!

Is this a low-fat diet?

No. A lot of research has been done on fats and most experts now agree that it isn't the overall quantity that counts but the quality and type of fat we eat. Kick the hydrogenated/trans fats into touch, keep saturated fats to a minimum and bring out the olive oil. We recommend using olive oil and olive oil-based spreads to increase your intake of these good, heart-healthy monounsaturated fats. The information we give on controlling your portion sizes will automatically keep your total fat intake at a healthy level.

What about desserts?

The odd pudding or dessert won't hurt but keep to the GL guidelines – base it on fruit or a couple of scoops of ice cream for a treat. Forget sugary, highly processed desserts and have something healthy instead – a few grapes, apple slices and a bit of cheese hits the spot for us, or a nice melon and fruit salad.

How much weight will I lose in seven days?

We aren't into quick fixes, but after seven days on the plan – providing you don't cheat and you move about a bit more – you should lose 2–5lb. Some people lose more if they have a lot of weight to lose. Your weight loss will depend on lots of factors including your metabolism, genes, general health, age and activity level.

Do I have to weigh myself every day?

This can be a bit negative, to be honest, especially for women as their water retention varies so much depending on cyclical hormonal changes within the body. How you wish to keep track of your weight loss, though, is your choice. Weighing once a week or every two weeks is preferable, and don't forget to measure specific areas before you start and every week after that. There is an inch-loss monitoring chart on page 44, or on our website. You will be amazed at your rate of inch loss. Most people know the weight at which they feel most comfortable, so there is no need to aim for an unrealistic target.

How many GL per day is low?

Although we don't advocate getting bogged down with counting, if you need the extra reassurance 80 GL per day would be classed as low and over 120 GL would be classed as high. Obviously the number of GL you can eat and lose weight will depend on many factors including your age, gender and activity levels.

Is alcohol forbidden?

When you consume alcohol your body uses it as a preferential fuel, so you will have to burn it off first before you burn off any fat. Remembering that you are delaying fat burning whenever you indulge in alcohol may be enough to put you off!

You will lose weight far more easily and quickly if you don't drink alcohol. If you must indulge, red wine is probably the best choice as at least it does appear to offer some health benefits, but only an occasional glass! Think of alcohol as empty calories you can do without (guess our popularity has just sunk to an all-time low now … ah well!).

What affects the GL of food?

Apart from the composition of the ingredients, other factors influence a food's GL, such as the type and degree of processing. The way ingredients interact is another factor, which is why testing products is important. The ripeness of some fruits and vegetables can also affect the glycaemic response. Adding acidity such as lemon/lime juice or vinegar can lower the GL of a food. Some high-fibre ingredients slow down gastric emptying, which also reduces the GL.

Getting active – how important is it to losing weight?

Activities (we like that word – it's much nicer than 'exercise' and conjures up fun rather than torture!) is vitally important. No getting away from it – particularly if you are trying to lose weight. Increasing your activity level – and that means anything from walking the dog to running a marathon to clearing out the loft – will improve your health and kick start your weight loss. Even three brisk 10-minute walks per day can be hugely beneficial. Whatever you decide to do, enjoy it – make it fun. The rewards in your mental clarity and the way you look and feel will be massive.

I have a friend who eats loads of rubbishy food and is like a stick insect.

Well, yes, we all know them and aren't they lucky – or are they? Thin doesn't always mean healthy, and if needing to lose weight gets you on the road to healthy eating that can only be a good thing. Some people are blessed with a genetically high metabolic rate, which means they will always be slim. The vast majority of us have a genetic predisposition to retain fat. This means that had we lived hundreds of years ago we would have survived in times of drought and famine! Now that food is more readily available, storing fat for future famines is no longer the benefit it once was.

Do I need to take nutritional supplements?

Foods are not as nutritious today as they once were due to depleted minerals in the soil as well as intensive farming methods, so a good-quality multivitamin and mineral supplement can be a worthwhile insurance policy.

How does a low-GL diet help control hunger?

Low-GL foods have a slower rate of absorption, which means that they reach the lower part of the small intestine, stimulating a feeling of fullness. Low-GL foods are more filling and delay hunger pangs for longer, which reduces food intake. When glucose levels go up and down after a high-GL meal, stress hormones such as cortisol and adrenalin are released, which stimulate appetite.

Can an underactive thyroid problem make it harder to lose weight?

This can often be the case. A shortage of thyroid hormone can reduce your body temperature and your metabolic rate. This can make you feel tired and less likely to be active. If you think you may have a thyroid problem, have a look at www.thyroiduk.org, an informative charity website set up for sufferers.

Where can I get more advice?

We have very lively, active forums on our website, www.dietfreedom.co.uk, where you will find lots of fellow Diet Freedom Fighters, who enjoy a good chitchat and in the process help each other to reach their goals. We never cease to be amazed at the intelligence, insight and information (not to mention humour) that emanates from the forums, and would highly recommend you pay them a visit. All three of us post in the forums regularly and offer help and support wherever we can. The website will also keep you up to speed with what we are up to at Diet Freedom HQ. We are currently very busy perfecting our range of Diet Freedom low-GL 'healthy treat' products – very exciting times!

Appendix 1

A–Z OF LOW-GL FOODS

For those who prefer to search alphabetically we have created a condensed A–Z list of low-GL foods. Do read through the 'main' food list in Chapter 10 thoroughly first, as it contains much more detailed information.

As GI/GL testing is ongoing, we aim to give you the most up-to-date information available, so any newly tested foods after publication of this book can be found on our website.

PLEASE NOTE: If foods are normally eaten cooked, the weights given are cooked weights, unless otherwise stated.

A

	Average portion	GL
Amaranth – 30g popped with milk has been tested as 21 so high-GL		
Anchovies*	120–150g	0
Apple juice	125ml	6
Arrabiata sauce	2–3 tbsp	NT
Artichoke	80g	0
Asparagus	80g	0

	Average portion	GL
Aubergine (eggplant)	80g	0
Avocado	80g	0
Avocado, mint and lime dressing	1 tbsp	NT

B

	Average portion	GL
Baked beans	80g	4
Balti sauce	2–3 tbsp	NT
Banana (green – under-ripe)	60g	3
Banana (yellow and green)	60g	6
Banana (ripe)	60g	7
Bean sprouts	80g	NT
Beef	75–120g	0
Beetroot	80g	4
Black-eyed beans	80g	5
Black pepper sauce	2–3 tbsp	NT
Blackberries	120g	0
Blueberries	120g	0
Bolognese sauce	2–3 tbsp	NT
Bran sticks	30g	NT
Broad beans	80g	5
Broccoli	80g	0
Brown rice	75g	9
Brussels sprouts	80g	0
Buckwheat kasha (boiled)	100g	10
Bulgur wheat (boiled)	100g	8
Butter	20g	0
Butter beans	80g	3

	Average portion	GL
C		
Cabbage	80g	0
Caesar dressing	1 tbsp	NT
Carrot juice	125ml	5
Carrots	80g	2
Cashew nuts	50g	3
Cauliflower	80g	0
Caviar	1 tbsp	0
Celeriac	80g	0
Celery	80g	0
Chana dal	80g	2
Chasseur sauce	2–3 tbsp	NT
Cheese – all types	50–75g	0
Cheese and chive dip	1 tbsp	NT
Cheese and onion dip	1 tbsp	NT
Cheese sauce	2–3 tbsp	NT
Cherries	120g	3
Chicken	100–150g	0
Chickpeas	80g	4
Chicory	80g	0
Chilli dressing	1 tbsp	NT
Chocolate – choose chocolate containing at least 70 per cent cocoa. A few squares as a snack is a great healthy choice!		
Coffee – be aware that some coffee bar chains add syrups to their coffees which will make them high-GL – ask for plain coffee or a cappuccino.		
Coleslaw	1 tbsp	0

	Average portion	GL
Collard greens	80g	0
Courgettes (zucchini)	80g	0
Couscous	100g	7
Cranberry juice	125ml	8
Cream	1 tbsp	NT
Crème fraîche	2 tbsp	NT
Cucumber	80g	0

D

Dark Swiss rye bread	30g	9
Diet drinks	1 can/bottle	NT
Dried apple	60g	10
Dried apricot	60g	9
Dried cranberries/mango/pineapple/ raspberries/strawberries	60g	NT
Dried prunes	60g	6
Duck	100–150g	0

E

Eggs	1	0
Endive	80g	0

F

Falafel	100g	NT
Fettuccine, egg	100g	10
Figs (fresh)	120g	NT
Flax seeds	50g	NT
Forestière sauce	2–3 tbsp	NT
French dressing	1 tbsp	NT

	Average portion	GL
Fructose	10g	2
Fruit tea	unlimited	NT

G

	Average portion	GL
Game	100–150g	0
Garlic and herb dip	1 tbsp	NT
Goat's milk (175ml/⅓ pint per day if used instead of cow's milk)	125ml	NT
Grapefruit	120g	3
Grapefruit juice	125ml	6
Grapes – black	120g	10
Grapes – green	120g	8
Guacamole	1 tbsp	NT

H

	Average portion	GL
Haricot (navy) beans	80g	6
Hazelnuts	50g	NT
Hemp seeds	50g	NT
Herbal tea	unlimited	NT
Herrings*	120–150g	0
Honey	25g	10
Honey and mustard dressing	1 tbsp	NT
Houmous	100g	<1

I

	Average portion	GL
Ice cream	50g	3–8

	Average portion	GL
J		
Jalfrezi sauce	2–3 tbsp	NT
Jam (jelly), reduced sugar	30g	5

	Average portion	GL
K		
Kale	80g	0
Kidney	75–120g	0
Kidney beans	80g	5
Kippers*	120–150g	0
Kiwis	120g	6
Kohlrabi	80g	0
Korma sauce	2–3 tbsp	NT

	Average portion	GL
L		
Lamb	75–120g	0
Leeks	80g	0
Lemons	1	0
Lentils	80g	3
Lettuce (all types)	80g	0
Lima beans	80g	5
Limes	1	0
Linseeds	50g	NT
Liver	75–120g	0

	Average portion	GL
M		
Macadamia nuts	50g	NT
Mackerel*	120–150g	0
Madeira sauce	2–3 tbsp	NT
Madras sauce	2–3 tbsp	NT

	Average portion	GL
Mandarins	120g	NT
Mange tout	80g	0
Mangoes	120g	8
Maple syrup	25g	9
Mayonnaise	1 tbsp	NT
Melons	120g	4
Milk, cow's (175ml/⅓ pint per day)	125ml	2
Muesli	30g	7–16
Mung bean noodles, dried	100g	8
Mung beans	80g	5
Mushroom sauce	2–3 tbsp	NT
Mushrooms	80g	0

N

Napoletana sauce	2–3 tbsp	NT
Nectarines	120g	NT

O

Oat bran (raw)	10g	3
Oat bran and honey bread	30g	7
Oatcakes	30g	8
Okra	80g	0
Olive oil	1 tbsp	0
Olive oil-based spread	20g	0
Olives	80g	0
Onions	80g	0
Orange juice	125ml	5
Oranges	120g	5
Ostrich	100–150g	0

	Average portion	GL
P		
Papaya (pawpaw)	120g	9–10
Parsnips (use sparingly)	80g	12
Peaches	120g	5
Peanuts	50g	1
Pearl barley	100g	5
Pears	120g	4
Peas	80g	3
Peas (marrowfat)	80g	4
Peas (split yellow)	80g	3
Pecans	50g	NT
Peppers	80g	0
Pesto sauce	2–3 tbsp	NT
Pilchards*	120–150g	0
Pine nuts	50g	NT
Pineapple juice	125ml	8
Pineapples	120g	7
Pinto beans	80g	5
Pistachio nuts	50g	NT
Plums	120g	5
Pomegranate juice	125ml	NT
Popcorn (plain, microwaved)	20g	8
Pork	75–120g	0
Porridge oats (steel-cut, cooked in water)	30g (dry weight)	9
Potatoes (baby new)	80g	6
Prunes (pitted)	60g	10
Pumpernickel bread	30g	5
Pumpkin	80g	3
Pumpkin seeds	50g	NT

	Average portion	GL
Puttanesca sauce	2–3 tbsp	NT

Q

	Average portion	GL
Quinoa	30g (dry weight)	9
Quorn	100–150g	NT

R

	Average portion	GL
Radicchio	80g	0
Radishes	80g	0
Raspberries	120g	0
Ravioli	100g	8
Red pepper dressing	1 tbsp	NT
Red wine and herb sauces	2–3 tbsp	NT
Rhubarb	120g	0
Rice bran, extruded	30g	3
Rice noodles	100g	10
Roasted vegetable sauces	2–3 tbsp	NT
Runner beans	80g	0
Rye (whole)	30g (dry weight)	8
Rye crackers	30g	10

S

	Average portion	GL
Salmon* (canned or fresh)	120–150g	0
Sardines*	120–150g	0
Sauerkraut	80g	0
Sausages	75–120g	0
Semolina (steamed)	100g	4
Sheep's milk (175ml/⅓ pint per day if used instead of cow's milk)	125ml	NT

	Average portion	GL
Shellfish	120–150g	0
Soba (buckwheat) noodles	100g	NT
Sour cream	1 tbsp	0
Sour cream and chive dip	1 tbsp	NT
Sourdough rye bread	30g	6
Soya (meat alternative)	100–150g	NT
Soya and linseed bread	30g	3
Soya beans	80g	<1
Soya milk (175ml/⅓ pint per day if used instead of cow's milk)	125ml	2
Soya yoghurt	100g	6
Spaghetti, white	100g	10
Spaghetti, wholemeal	100g	9
Spelt hasn't been individually tested so use sparingly for now.		
Spelt multigrain bread	30g	7
Spinach	80g	0
Spinach and ricotta or nutmeg sauce	2–3 tbsp	NT
Spring onions (scallions)	80g	0
Squash (all)	80g	0
Strawberries	120g	1
Sunflower and barley bread	30g	6
Sunflower seeds	50g	NT
Swede	80g	7
Sweet pepper sauce	2–3 tbsp	NT
Sweet potatoes	80g	9
Sweetcorn	80g	9
Swiss chard	80g	0

	Average portion	GL
T		
Tabbouleh	50g	NT
Tangerines	120g	NT
Tarragon sauce	2–3 tbsp	NT
Tea (black/green)	unlimited	NT
Tikka masala sauce	2–3 tbsp	NT
Tomato and basil dressing	1 tbsp	NT
Tomato and basil sauce	2–3 tbsp	NT
Tomato and mascarpone sauce	2–3 tbsp	NT
Tomato and roasted onion dressing	1 tbsp	NT
Tomato juice	125ml	2
Tomato salsa	1 tbsp	NT
Tomatoes	80g	0
Tortellini, cheese	100g	6
Tuna*	120–150g	0
Turkey	100–150g	0
Turnips	80g	0
Tzatziki	1 tbsp	NT

U		
Ugli fruit	120g	NT

V		
Vinaigrette dressing	1 tbsp	NT

W		
Walnuts	50g	NT
Watercress	80g	0
Watercress sauce	2–3 tbsp	NT

	Average portion	GL
Watermelon	120g	4
Wheat (whole)	30g (dry weight)	8
White fish	150–200g	0
White wine sauce	2–3 tbsp	NT
Wholegrain bread	30g	7
Wholemeal pitta bread	30g	10
Wholemeal rye bread	30g	8
Wild rice	75g	8

Y

	Average portion	GL
Yams	80g	7
Yoghurt	200g	2–4
Yoghurt and mint dressing	1 tbsp	NT
Yoghurt drinks (sugar-free)	1 standard size	NT

denotes oily fish

RECOMMENDED READING

Brand-Miller, Professor Jennie. *The New Glucose Revolution*, Marlowe & Company, 2004

Collier, Roz and Foster, Georgia. *Slim by Suggestion*, HarperCollins, 2001

Denby, Nigel, van der Heijden, Tina and Pyner, Deborah. *The GL Diet*, John Blake, 2004

Denby, Nigel and Baic, Sue. *Nutrition for Dummies*, Whiley, 2005

The Mind Gym, Time Warner, 2005

Roth, Sally. *The Modern Herb Gardener*, Carroll & Brown, 2001

Willett, Dr Walter C. *Eat, Drink, and Be Healthy*, Simon & Schuster, 2004

We really hope you enjoyed reading this book and that you have found it useful. We'd love to hear your feedback at www.dietfreedom.co.uk

Nigel, Tina and Deborah

xxx

Index

A-Z food list 297–308
Acidity 293
activities 15, 18–23, 40, 52–7, 243, 290, 292, 294
advice 37, 296
al dente 207
alcohol 51, 241, 293
almond oil 257
amaranth 248
American Journal of Clinical Nutrition 275, 277–9, 288
American Journal of Epidemiology 286–7
antioxidants 195, 245, 249–50, 260
Archives of Gynaecology 276
Archives of Pediatric and Adolescent Medicine 276
arrowroot 188
arteries 194, 277
arthritis 278
asthma 278
Australia 4, 281
avocado oil 257
Aztecs 248

barley 208, 244, 247–8, 282

beans 194, 198, 207–8, 236, 249, 267, 282
berries 192, 199–200, 266, 285
binge drinking 51
biscuits 49–51, 239, 256–7, 263, 290
blood glucose/sugar 5–6, 9–10
  food lists 192, 211
  guides 63, 77, 109, 188
  motivation 51
  questions 289–90, 295
  research 278, 284, 287
blood pressure 43, 55, 262
Body Mass Index (BMI) 14, 39, 42–3, 276, 286–7
boredom 10, 36, 290
bran 244–5, 250–2
Brand-Miller, Jennie 286
bread 8–9, 51, 187–8, 206, 242
  lifestyle 247, 253
  research 278, 280–1, 284–5
breakfast 16, 62, 64, 78
  guides 107, 110
  lifestyle 193, 250, 253, 266
  research 278, 281, 284

breastfeeding 255, 268
breathing rate 23
Brigham and Women's Hospital 284, 286
British Journal of Nutrition 279, 287
buckwheat 156, 188, 248–9
buffets 241
bulgur wheat 247, 249
bust measurements 40, 44
butchers 239–40

C-reactive protein (CRP) 277–8, 285
calcium 261, 267
calorie counting 290
Canada 4, 280
cancer 41, 43, 55, 201, 246, 280
Cancer Council 281
canned foods *see* tinned foods
canteens 62
car washing 56
carbohydrates 3–4, 7–10, 192, 199, 204, 277–9, 281–9
cereals 193, 244–53, 278, 284
chair exercises 56
chest measurements 40, 44
Children's Hospital Boston 284, 288
chilli 107–8, 145
chocolate 209
cholesterol 43, 245, 249–50, 256, 277, 280
coconut oil 258
coffee 209, 242, 265

complacency 49–50
confidence 46–7
constipation 245, 264
convenience foods 234–7
corn 249–50
crackers 206, 239
cravings 6, 62, 191
cupped-hands portion guide 14, 191, 242
cycling 54

dairy foods 194, 201–3, 256, 261, 266–7
dancing 54
dehydration 264–5
deli counters 236
desserts 51, 236, 241, 291
diabetes 41, 43–4, 50, 55
  lifestyle 246
  research 275–7, 280–1, 283, 285–6
Diabetes Care 275, 281
Diet Freedom Fighters
  guides 145
  motivation 37, 47
  questions 290, 296
  role 12, 15, 26
  temptation 50
diet trap 3, 27–8, 30, 33, 49, 51
digging 56
dinner 65, 79, 111
dinner-party foods 240–1
dips 211, 213
disease 41, 43–4, 50, 55
  lifestyle 201, 245–6, 254, 256, 262

research 277–8, 280, 282,
   285–6, 288
doctors 20, 40, 56, 268
dressings 211, 214, 257–60
dried fruit 200–1, 267
drinks 37, 209–10, 240–1,
   264–8

eating disorders 52
eating out 17, 34, 37, 49,
   74–5, 217, 240–2
eating plans 16–18, 33, 35–6,
   38, 290–1
Edward I 248
eggs 194, 202, 266–7
endorphins 55
endosperm 244, 252
energy 53, 268
essential oils 257–61
evening meals 16–17
evening primrose oil 260
exercise 5, 52–3, 56, 265,
   294

family meals 37
famine 294
FAQs 289–96
farmers' markets 239
farming 295
fast foods 242
Fast and Friendly Plan 16–17,
   61–75, 218–22
fat intake 243, 253–61,
   283–4, 288, 290–1
fats 5–6, 19, 40, 44, 54, 268,
   270
fibre 198, 206, 209, 244–5

lifestyle 249, 252–3, 268,
   276, 286
questions 293
research 276, 286
fish 194–5, 214, 235, 241–2,
   254–5, 263, 266–7
fish oils 254–5
fishmongers 239–40
fitness classes 54
flavanols 209
flax oil 260
flours 187–8, 239, 247, 287
fluids 43, 243
Food and Agriculture
   Organization (FAO) 286
food groups 4, 16, 266
food lists 12–13, 35, 37,
   191–216, 247, 290
Foodie Friendly Plan 18,
   107–44, 228–34
forums 23, 37, 47, 146, 296
Frost, Gary 287
fructose 188, 210–11
fruit 199–201, 209, 236, 284
   lifestyle 242–3, 246, 266–7
   questions 291, 293
frying 258, 260

game 193
gardening 108
garlic 76–7, 107, 145
germ 244–5, 250–1
gluten-free foods 156, 206–7,
   248, 251
Glycaemic Index (GI) 3–11
Glycaemic Load (GL) 3–11
goal-setting 39–47

grains 205, 239, 244–53, 267, 287
groundnut oil 259
guilt 27, 29, 49
gut bacteria 245–6

Hammersmith Hospitals NHS Trust 287
Harvard Medical School 4, 10, 286
hazelnut oil 259
health 43, 53, 201, 209, 234
  lifestyle 244–5, 253, 256, 262–3, 269–70
  questions 292–4
  research 281
health-food stores 239
healthy treats 296
heart 19, 41, 43–4, 50, 54–5
  lifestyle 201, 246, 254, 256, 262
  questions 291
  research 277, 280, 282, 286, 288
help 37
hempseed oil 259
herbs 76–7, 107–8, 186, 215, 237
high-glycaemic foods 5–7, 13, 36
high-street shops 239–40
hip measurements 40, 44
Hodge, Alison 281
hormones 5, 55, 295
housework 55
hunger pangs 13, 36, 246, 284, 295

hydrogenated fats 201, 208, 243, 256, 291

immunity 55
Incas 251
insulin 5, 277, 282–5
International Journal of Obesity 277
Internet shopping 238
Inuit 254
irritability 51

jams/jellies 210, 239
Japanese 254
jars 236–7
Journal of the American Medical Association 276, 282–3
Journal of the National Cancer Institute 280
juices 209, 266

labels 235, 247, 250, 256, 262, 268–70
Lancet 280
lapses 48–51
lauric acid 258
lemon juice 108
lifestyle 12–13, 15, 52, 245
lime juice 108
liver 5
low-fat foods 269
low-glycaemic foods 5–8, 12, 37, 191–216, 234–7, 297–308
low-sugar foods 270
Ludwig, David 278, 284–5, 288

lunch 16, 35, 48, 55, 65
 guides 72–3, 78, 107, 110
 lifestyle 192
 research 281

meals 13, 16, 35, 37, 49
 guides 62, 107
 lifestyle 218, 263
 research 284
measurements 14, 40, 42–7
meat 193–4, 235, 241–2,
 256, 263, 266
memory 55
men 63, 77, 109
mercury 255
metabolic rate 19, 54, 192,
 283, 294–5
milk 261
minerals 195, 295
mobility 56
monounsaturated fats 243,
 254, 291
mood swings 51
motivation 41, 43–4, 47
mowing 56
muscles 5, 40, 54

no-added-sugar foods 270
noodles 207, 239
nutrition 13, 16, 34, 192
 lifestyle 243–5, 266, 268
 questions 295
 research 283
nuts 194, 203–4, 239, 267,
 284, 287, 290

oats 188, 244, 247, 250, 285

oils 167, 201–3, 237, 256–61
olive oil 258, 260–1, 291
omega-3 fats 194, 254–5,
 258–9
omega-6 fats 258–9
omega-9 fats 257, 259
Optimal Weight for Life (OWL)
 284
optimism 46–7
organic foods 193, 239
organization 14

pancreas 5
pasta 207, 235, 239, 242, 247,
 253
pâtés 214
Pediatrics 278, 281
Pereira, Mark 283
physiotherapy 56
phytoestrogens 245
planning 34–6, 41, 217
polyols 210
polyunsaturated fats 243,
 254
portion guidelines 247
portion size 8, 10, 14, 37,
 191–216, 278, 291
potatoes 235, 242, 278
poultry 193, 235
pre-packaged meals 235
pregnancy 255, 268, 276, 279
processed foods 188, 234–7,
 243, 263, 291, 293
protein 4, 194, 248–9, 251–3,
 261, 267–8, 283
pulses 194, 198, 207–8, 236
pumpkin oil 260

questionnaire 30–2
quinoa 251
Quorn 194, 239

ready-made foods 17, 235–7,
    262–3
recipes 12, 35–6, 206, 208
reduced-fat foods 269
reduced-sugar foods 270
refined foods 188, 244–6,
    251, 284, 286–7
relapses 48–51
research 8–11, 275–88
restaurants 37, 50, 240, 242
rice 208, 235–6, 242, 244,
    251, 278, 280
rice-bran oil 260
roller-blading 54
80/20 rule 52, 241
rutin 249
rye 187–8, 244, 252

saboteurs 38
salad leaves 108
salt 243, 262–3
saturated fats 201, 254, 256,
    291
sauces 211–13, 235–6, 242,
    262–3
scales 14, 43, 45
seeds 203–4, 239, 267, 287
sesame oil 259
Seven-Day GL Diet 12–26
sex 55–6
shopping guides 12–13, 34–5,
    217–42
skipping 55

sleep 19, 55
Smiley Face Score 45–6
smoothies 209, 242
snacks 13, 16, 35–6, 48, 62
    guides 64–5, 73–4, 77–9,
        110–11
    lifestyle 209, 240, 262–3
soil 295
soya 194, 203, 239, 261,
    267–8
spelt 156, 187–8, 252
spices 107–8, 215, 237
spikes 5
spreads 201, 256, 291
starters 241–2
stress 19, 27, 295
stroke 286
subconscious 38
sugars 210–11, 213, 235–6,
    242, 268–70, 279, 284,
    290
sunflower oil 258–9
supplements 268, 295
support 38–9
sweeteners 210–11
swimming 54, 56

talk test 23
tape measures 40
temptation 50–1, 238
testing 9, 289, 293
thyroid 295
tinned foods 201, 236, 255,
    263, 267
trampolining 55
trans fatty acids (TFAs) 201,
    208, 256–7, 291

treats 296
triglycerides 256, 277, 280, 285

United States 4
University of Massachusetts Medical School (UMMS) 286–7
University of Minnesota 283
University of Sydney 4
University of Toronto 4, 280

vegans 266, 268
vegetables 195–7, 208, 236
  lifestyle 239, 242–3, 246, 266–7
  questions 293
  research 284, 287
vegetarians 17, 33, 76–105, 194, 223, 255, 266
Veggie Friendly Plan 17, 76–106, 223–8, 266
vinegars 167
virgin oils 258
vitamins 195, 245, 257, 260–1, 266, 268, 295

waist measurements 40, 44
waiters 241
walking 19–23, 54–5, 290, 294
walnut oil 259
water 209, 240–1, 243, 264–8, 292
websites 16, 23, 39, 47, 145, 192, 289, 292, 295–6
weighing 10, 292
weight control 5–7, 51–3
weight-for-height charts 39
wheat 244, 252–3
wholegrains 244–53, 267, 284
wild rice 253
Willett, Walter 10, 286
willpower 27, 49
women 63, 77, 109
World Health Organization (WHO) 286

xanthan gum 188

yoghurt drinks 209–10, 242
Yunsheng Ma 287

Index of Recipes

Andie's Greek chicken 146–7
apricot jam 175
asparagus, lemon and mint
    barleyotto 92–3
avocado
    and butterbean salad 102–3
    herby guacamole 114
    and prawns 66
    tomato, mozzarella and
        spinach salad 95
    and tomato pot 97

bacon
    and bean salad 162–3
    quinoa and rocket salad with
        warm dressing 160–1
baked sweet potato with
    cheese and tomato 83
banana, mint and raspberry
    yoghurt with toasted seeds
    180
barley
    asparagus, lemon and mint
        barleyotto 92–3
    basic barleyotto 154
    prawn, asparagus and pea
        barleyotto 155

red pepper, chorizo and basil
    barleyotto 134–5
barleyotto 154
beans
    and bacon salad 162–3
    butterbean and avocado salad
        102–3
    chunky bacon soup 128–9
    mixed salad 82
    nutty chickpea and sesame
        burgers 86
    roasted vegetable and bulgur
        wheat salad 132–3
    spicy bulgur wheat and butter
        bean 84–5
    sprout salad 94
beef
    fast fettuccine Bolognese 69
    and vegetable casserole 138–9
blackberry and apple crumble
    176–7
bread, nutty seedy 116–17
bulgur wheat and butter bean
    salad 84–5
butterbean and avocado salad
    with heavenly grilled pepper
    dressing 102–3

butternut squash, curried
90–1

cake, outrageously indulgent
celebration 184–5
carrot and coriander mash 171
casserole, beef and vegetable
138–9
cauliflower
mash with grainy mustard and
Parmesan 169
and tomato crumble 104–5
celeriac mash with spring
onions and chives 170
chicken
Andie's Greek 146–7
breasts with blue cheese and
watercress 148
chilli, lime and ginger 127
drunken gin and juniper roast
182–3
lemon and herb barleyotto
155
roast 182–3
spicy peanut 149
spicy salad 67
chickpeas
houmous 142
and pepper salad 124
and sesame burgers 86
zesty vegetable kebabs
88–9
chilli
lime and garlic spinach 173
lime and ginger chicken 127
chorizo, red pepper and basil
barleyotto 134–5

chunky bean and bacon soup
128–9
courgette, garlic and basil pasta
98–9
creamy dishes
cauliflower mash with
grainy mustard and
Parmesan 169
olive tapenade dressing 166
curried butternut squash
90–1

desserts
apricot jam 175
blackberry and apple crumble
176–7
strawberry and fresh fig
brûlée 178
Diet Freedom
muesli 112–13
toasted seed mix 121
dips
herby cream cheese 137
houmous 142
mucho-spicy 143
raita 130
tzatziki 130
dressings
all-round blend 168
creamy olive tapenade 166
heavenly grilled pepper
102–3
herby oils/vinegars 167
warm 160–1
warm toasted sesame 165
drunken gin and juniper roast
chicken 182–3

fast fettuccine Bolognese 69
feta cheese, marinated 115
fish
  giant prawns with mucho-
    spicy dip 143
  grilled hoki with rocket
    and sun-dried tomato salad
    131
  grilled mackerel and cheese
    on toast 153
  haddock with spinach,
    mushrooms and crème
    fraîche 152
  pan-fried tuna steaks with
    tomato sauce 68
  salmon pesto 71
  scrambled eggs with smoked
    salmon 141
  smoked mackerel pâté 126
  spicy chilli prawns 151
  tuna steaks with tomato and
    basil sauce 118–19
French bean salad 159

giant prawns with mucho-spicy
  dip 143
goat's cheese with pear 136
Greek dishes
  salad 70
  yoghurt with nuts, seeds, mint
    and fresh ginger 136
grilled dishes
  hoki with rocket and sun-
    dried tomato salad 131
  mackerel and cheese on toast
    153
guacamole 114

haddock with spinach,
  mushrooms and crème
  fraîche 152
heavenly grilled pepper
  dressing 102–3
herbs
  butter 186
  cream cheese 137
  guacamole 114
  vinegar 186
hoki with rocket and sun-dried
  tomato salad 131
houmous 142

kebabs, zesty vegetable 88–9

lemon
  chicken and herb barleyotto
    155
  heaven 96
lentil and tomato salad 87
lunch box ideas 72–3

mackerel
  and cheese on toast 153
  pâté 126
marinades
  all-round blend 168
  feta cheese 115
mashes
  carrot and coriander 171
  celeriac with spring onions
    and chives 170
  creamy cauliflower with grainy
    mustard and Parmesan 169
melon
  and mint fruit salad 125

and mint with halloumi cheese
164
minty yoghurt, sugar snap and
sun-dried tomato pasta
sauce 157
muesli 112–13
mushrooms on low-GL toast
100

nuts
chickpea and sesame burgers
86
seedy bread 116–17

outrageously indulgent
celebration cake 184–5

pan-fried tuna steaks with
tomato sauce 68
pasta
minty yoghurt, sugar snap
and sun-dried tomato 157
perfect 156
toasted courgette, garlic and
basil 98–9
variations 158
pea and mint soup 140
perfect pasta 156
pesto salmon 71
porridge 80
prawns
asparagus and pea barleyotto
155
with mucho-spicy dip 143
spicy chilli 151

raita 130

red pepper, chorizo and basil
barleyotto 134–5
roast dishes
Sunday lunch 181
tomatoes 174
vegetable, bean and bulgur
wheat salad 132–3

salads
avocado, tomato, mozzarella
and spinach 95
bacon and bean 162–3
bacon, quinoa and rocket
160–1
bean 82
bean sprout 94
Bisbas 81
chickpea and pepper 124
Greek 70
grilled hoki with rocket and
sun-dried tomato 131
lentil and tomato 87
melon and mint fruit 125
melon and mint with halloumi
cheese 164
roasted vegetable, bean and
bulgur wheat 132–3
spicy bulgur wheat and butter
bean 84–5
spicy chicken 67
warm French bean 159
salmon, pesto 71
sauces
minty yoghurt, sugar snap
and sun-dried tomato 157
tomato 122–3
tomato and basil 118–19

scrambled eggs with smoked
   salmon 141
smoked mackerel pâté 126
snack ideas 73–4
soups
   chunky bean and bacon
      128–9
   pea and mint 140
   tomato, garlic and basil 150
spicy dishes
   bulgur wheat and butter bean
      salad 84–5
   chicken salad 67
   chilli prawns 151
   meatballs with tomato sauce
      122–3
   peanut chicken 149
squash, curried 90–1
strawberry and fresh fig brûlée
   178
summer berries with Greek
   yoghurt 120
sweet potato, baked with
   cheese and tomato 83

toasted dishes
   courgette, garlic and basil
      pasta 98–9
   seed mix 121
tomato
   and basil sauce 118–19
   and cauli crumble 104–5
   garlic and basil soup 150
   sauce 122–3
tuna
   pan-fried steaks with tomato
      sauce 68

steaks with tomato and basil
   sauce 118–19
tzatziki 130

vanilla and blueberry yoghurt
   179
vegetables
   bean and bulgur wheat salad
      132–3
   beef casserole 138–9
   chilli, lime and garlic spinach
      173
   Greek style 101
   kebabs with wild rice 88–9
   roasted tomatoes 174
   zingy new potatoes 172
veggie mashes
   carrot and coriander mash
      171
   celeriac with spring onions
      and chives 170
   creamy cauliflower with grainy
      mustard and Parmesan 169

warm dishes
   dressing 160–1
   French bean salad 159
   toasted sesame dressing 165

yoghurt
   banana, mint and raspberry
      180
   vanilla and blueberry 179

zesty vegetable kebabs with wild
   rice and chickpeas 88–9
zingy new potatoes 172